Books by Cynthia Olsen

Australian Tea Tree Oil Guide (1st ed.)

Australian Tea Tree Oil Guide (2nd ed.)

Australian Tea Tree Oil Handbook:
101 Ways to Use Australian Tea Tree Oil (1st ed.)

Australian Tea Tree Oil Handbook:
101 Plus Ways to Use Australian Tea Tree Oil (2nd ed.)

Essiac: A Native Herbal Cancer Remedy (2nd ed.)

Birth of the Blue: Australian Blue Cypress Oil

Looking Up:

Seven Steps *for a* Healthy & Youthful Midlife *and* Beyond

Dedication

I dedicate this book to my grandparents and parents who were my outstand-ing teachers and who instilled in me core values which have sustained me throughout my lifetime.

To my sister Patricia, a guiding force who left us too soon.

To the next generation, my children and grandchildren, my love for you is everlasting. My wish for you, long and healthy lives.

To my great nephew Joe who has taught our family the true meaning of love. His attitude of gratitude has given him the ability to conquer his limitations.

To Sharon and Bob - God bless you.

I also dedicate this book to the fellowship of my far reaching extended family that has1touched my life with love, support and encouragement.

To all of you I am eternally grateful.

Page & Cover Design/Cover Art: Paul Bond
Editors: Anne Barthel, Susan Tinkle & Lynn Kelley

Manufactured in the United States of America

Published by Kali Press
PO Box 5491, Eagle, Colorado 81631

10 9 8 7 6 5 4 3 2 1
First Edition

Looking Up: Seven Steps for a Healthy & Youthful Midlife and Beyond

Disclaimer
This book is educational in nature and is not be used for medical diagnosis or treatment. This book is not intended to substitute for medical care by a licensed health care professional. Treatment of individual health problems must be closely supervised by a physician. The author recommends against changing any current medication, altering current therapy, or adding new therapies without first consulting a physician.

Kali Press
Eagle, Colorado

Table of Contents

Foreword

C. Norman Shealy, M.D., Ph.D.

Considering my observations in working with over 30,000 patients and talking to many more, I believe virtually everyone needs to build a healthy and more youthful life. Forty percent of us in this country are clinically depressed and another forty percent have what I call sub-clinical depressive miasma. Even though twenty percent have somehow escaped the cloud of depression, only three percent have all of the essential four habits for healthy living:

- No smoking
- Body Mass Index of 18 to 24
- Minimum of 5 servings of fruits or veggies daily
- Exercise 30 minutes or more 5 days a week

And that list does not even include sleep! A majority of us do not sleep the required seven or eight hours each night. In this book, Cynthia suggests concrete steps you can take toward a life with (and I apologize for my simplification of her common-sense approach):

- An optimal attitude
- Exercise
- Nutrition
- Supplements
- Attention to total body care

- Financial common sense
- Living in the Now

That, folks, is a major step forward!! For around ninety-seven percent of Americans it requires far more purposeful will power than has been obvious in the past five thousand years. For at least forty years I have asked countless thousands of people why they do not care about health! It seems so obvious to me---nothing is more important than personal health. Without optimal health, you cannot optimize anything in your life. Yes, I believe the only real purpose in life is to help others. But if you neglect helping yourself first, then you have far less to offer others.

I realize that for five thousand years women in many societies have been put down—pure insanity! And for two thousand years churches have taught that we are all sinners, born in sin. What utter nonsense. But just a little common sense tells us that those two concepts put forth by the power-crazy despots who wish to control everyone (except themselves!), are without merit. If you have enough self-esteem to say "I'm OK, because God does not create junk," then you are ready to use Looking Up: Seven Steps for a Healthy & Youthful Midlife and Beyond. This book is an important first step towards living a conscious, conscientious life.

Norman Shealy, M.D., Ph.D. is president of Holos Institutes of Health, Professor Emeritus of Energy Medicine, Holos University Graduate Seminary and Founding President, American Holistic Medical Association. He has au-thored over 300 articles and 28 books, including Life Beyond 100: Medical Intuition & Energy Medicine.

www.normshealy.com
www.medicalrenaissance.net
www.holosinstitutesofhealth.com
www.holosuniversity.org

Introduction

"Wake up! If you knew for certain you had a terminal illness... if you had little time left to live – you would waste precious little of it! Well, I'm telling you... you do have a terminal illness. It's called birth. You don't have more than a few years left. No one does. So be happy now, without reason – or you will never be at all."

~"THE WAY OF THE PEACEFUL WARRIOR," DAN MILLMAN

*W*hen you have your health, you have everything," my grandmother Jennie used to tell me when I was growing up. She should know, having lost a leg to Diabetes Mellitus Type 2 in her 60's and then learning to walk again in spite of all the adversities. She would repeat the phrase quite often; perhaps it became the mantra that gave her courage and strength to get up each morning, put on her prosthesis, and go about her daily life. She survived into her upper 70's, passing away in her sleep. Her resilience and attitude, coupled with faith in herself and God, gave her a longer life than the doctors predicted. She outlived her husband and one of her daughters, my mother.

I had a healthy start in my own life. I grew up in an Italian-American family with both maternal and paternal grandparents born in Italy, so I followed a Mediterranean diet long before it became *en vogue*. My mother prepared fresh, wholesome food, and what a difference fresh food makes. We always had a variety of yogurt, vegetables, dairy, and meat on hand. Milk was delivered in glass bottles with thick cream floating on the top. There were no genetically modified foods back then.

Sugar, however, was everywhere. During the holidays, we enjoyed luscious (and rich) Italian baked goods. Life was delicious. My grandmother

Jennie was addicted to sugar. She stashed sweets in a hideout in the pantry. When her diabetes got worse, I believe she regretted not having more will power to overcome her sugar addiction.

My parents were not physically active people, and as a result their health was compromised as they grew older, something I witnessed firsthand. My mother developed rheumatoid arthritis and my dad, kidney disease. My mother suffered ongoing aches in her 30's. Her hands and feet were so badly crippled she couldn't open a jar or fit her swollen feet into shoes. She spent many years depressed and in pain. My father looked after her, and the daily stress took a terrible toll on his well-being too.

As children, my siblings and I were careful to monitor our behavior based on whether my mother's bedroom door was closed during the day, indicating she was resting. My dad was always trying to compensate for my mother's forced inactivity by taking us on sojourns into the city or Sunday drives in the car. She had no desire to exercise or go to therapy—especially after falling and breaking her hip at age 45. Her medical doctor and the National Institute of Health wanted to run more extensive research on her because of her severe RA; however, she refused as she seemed to refuse taking more positive steps to improve her health. Some winter days my father would find her hanging clothes outside which would only make her joints swell and send her to bed. My mother tried to control everything around her. I read once that people who suffer with RA possess a rigid manner in their life. I often wondered if there was a correlation between that and my mother's RA. As far as we can determine, there hasn't been any other family member diagnosed with RA. After years of ill health, my mother developed lupus and died of a stroke at 53. I was 26 at the time. My dad passed away 6 weeks later, at 63; his death is still unexplained. I think he died of a broken heart.

* * * *

I have always thrived on being active—swimming at three, tennis, baseball, basketball, roller skating, hiking, canoeing, biking, horseback riding—you name it. So as I get older, it's been like second nature to incorporate more activity into my days. However, I was not yet sitting still long enough to rest; that was a challenge for me. In my 20's and halfway into my 30's, I was raising my five very active children, and I didn't yet know and understand the spiritual side of life. I had occasional flashes of insight and the feeling that there was a good deal more for me to learn about my spiritual side, but there was little time to contemplate these feelings while meeting the demands of my family.

Into my 30's I began to read books by Carlos Castaneda, a Peruvian author who wrote about his teacher, a Yaqui shaman named Don Juan Mateus, whom he met in 1960. The teacher taught him the ways of a Yaqui warrior. I expanded my yearnings for more in-depth spiritual knowledge through *The Prophet*, and explored psychic writings by Jane Roberts—*Seth Speaks*, among others. Jane was considered one of the leading psychics in the twentieth century. She would often go into a trance and write about her communications. She lived within an hour of us in upper New York State when I was 25. My friend was her neighbor and told me we could come to her place and participate in a spiritual meeting, but I was naïve at the time, and had little interest in meeting her. Perhaps it wasn't the time for me to explore this area even though the Ouija board became constant entertainment for us.

I quit smoking cigarettes when I was 28, before the Surgeon General's report on the hazards of tobacco. My sixth sense told me that inhaling tobacco would eventually compromise my health in some way. I also cut back on alcohol at around the same time, as the two habits seemed to go hand and hand.

My parents had the foresight to ship my siblings and me off to camp during the summer months. In the Adirondack Mountains, where I spent most of my early years, the air and lakes seemed especially clean during the 1950's. I swam in our lake along with the fish, turtles, and water plants. We didn't talk about global warming back then, nor did we see any evidence of pollution, although acid rain eventually destroyed most of the flora and fish. The days were bright and clear, and the evening sky was filled with a magnificent showing of the Northern Lights.

We were raised in the Catholic Church, but as I grew up I pulled away, seeking alternative spiritual avenues. I began to practice yoga when I was in my mid-30's and made friends who talked about metaphysics and what it meant to be psychic. I began to find ways to balance my days, to become more peaceful and to better handle stress. I lived in the Colorado Mountains and would seek out solitude through hikes into the wilderness areas. In the winter, I cross-country skied on trails away from the tourists. I cooked healthy foods, not unlike the Mediterranean diet I grew up with. I read every label on the supermarket shelves. I started to experiment with cooking tofu, and digging my hands into a garden of vegetables. I frequented farmers markets for fresh fruits and produce. I made healthy school lunches of organic peanut butter spread on luscious whole grain bread. My world back then seemed like a laboratory, with me as the mad chemist; everyone within my reach became my guinea pig.

I look back on that period of my life as my education in health, even though I wasn't totally conscious of it. I purchased healthy recipe cookbooks; *Laura's Kitchen* became my kitchen Bible. The children sometimes questioned what they were eating, but I persevered. My youngest step son wasn't used to eating healthy food and at dinner would run to the bathroom to throw up. I was extremely grateful that he didn't continue this ritual. Sometimes for desert I would bake a yummy cheesecake made with tofu and fresh fruit. At first they would express amazement that I made such a desert until they were told its ingredients. They seemed to be ok with the healthier version. Nutrition has been an ongoing journey in my life. Genetically modified foods (GMO), herbicides and pesticides, processed foods, hormone injected beef, chickens raised under unsanitary conditions, to name just a few, have invaded our planet since I grew into adulthood, so I became watchful in the types of food to prepare.

My many gardens were experimental. In the mountains I would haul my neighbor's animal manure down the road to prepare my garden for planting. My daughter's horse escaped one day and I had to chase him away before he ate all of the lettuce. During my 20's we lived in Southern Florida on an acre of land. I rented a Rototiller to prepare the garden. I was a novice so decided to plant radishes to begin with. In spring, we had a variety of red, white, and hot radishes growing amongst a few bunches of lettuce. The avocado, banana and mango trees on our property provided us with fresh fruit.

What I've learned from all the people and experiences I've had is that my life has always presented opportunities for me to have stepping stones to grow, and those simple changes, especially when presented in times of adversity, made a big difference. We are all born with a finite set of genes; but they are only one factor in our health among many— and the only one that we can't control in some way. I have walked the major avenues to longevity and vitality; nutrition, exercise, positive relationships, quality health care, geographic location, financial well-being, the mind-body connection, and avoiding alcohol, tobacco, and drugs. I want to pass along what I've learned so others can also be vibrant into their 50's, 60's, and beyond.

* * * *

A few weeks before taking a trip to the Bahamas in the summer of 2009, I thought back to my mother's deteriorating physical condition in 1968, and realized that I had no idea how she really felt about either her deteriorating health or the endless trips to the hospital and doctors. I could only imagine what it may have been like. It was a prophecy soon to be realized for me. I had not been in a hospital for 40 years, having worked hard to stay far from them.

The trip started out as a grand adventure with my daughter Kimberly, her husband Dan and two of my grandchildren Haley and Gavin, to an exotic, out-of-the-way South Andros Island in the Bahamas. The island people were poor so they relied on the general store. Food and sundries were delivered by boat from the mainland once a week. We were there during crab season when these gigantic crustaceans would crawl over the island to make their way back to the ocean. It was a huge hunting event for the locals. The beach house we rented was rustic but bright and clean. There was an old-fashioned screen porch which extended the length of the house. A hammock was at one end and the other had more beds for the kids to sleep. There was a rectangular wooden dining table and a smaller one for our nightly card games.

Beyond that were sparkling vistas of bleached white sand leading to a gazebo and miles of private beach. The turquoise color of the ocean was a perfect compliment for the sailfish and two ocean kayaks that were there for us to use at our leisure. A volleyball net was set up near the house and the owners' two island dogs kept us company.

On the third night of the trip, I was walking from the bathroom to retrieve a book when suddenly I tripped over a landing and catapulted in midair, flying directly toward the cement floor. The second I hit the floor I knew that I had done something horrific to my right arm. A bone protruded out. The family had heard me cry out and brought a first aid kit after lifting me up and placing me on a nearby chair. I sat—probably in shock—while they cleaned up my injury and prepared a makeshift splint. It was after midnight and the owner, who lived in an adjacent apartment, called the only doctor on the island. He was just a few miles down the road but the trip there felt like an eternity. The clinic was also the doctor's home. He was East Indian and spoke very little English. He undressed my wrapping and splint and poured a liquid onto the wrist which I imagine was some kind of disinfectant. Then he gave me a shot to reduce the risk of infection. The doctor told my daughter I needed to get the morning plane to Nassau to receive immediate care at Doctors Hospital, a private medical facility.

Kimberly and I took the flight while Dan stayed behind with the children. The Indian doctor appeared at the airport, wrote some notes for us to take to the hospital, and wished me well. It was a welcome, kind, and compassionate gesture from the island doctor after what seemed like an endless night of anxiety and pain.

My brother found out about my accident and came to my rescue buying me two plane tickets in order for me to get home. On the first leg I traveled from Nassau to Orlando, Florida where my brother and his wife met me, took me to lunch, and stayed for several hours until my plane left for Denver. I asked my brother to get a wheelchair to take me to the gate. The plane was full. When I arrived at the gate, I asked if there was a seat closer up. My ticket was for a seat at the back of the plane. I knew I wouldn't have the fortitude or desire to walk to that seat. Fortunately, there was one cancellation and I was able to sit in the third row. I traveled back to Colorado to face four surgeries at Vail Valley Medical Center and have hand therapies and endless exams by my orthopedic physician, at Steadman Philippon Research Institute in Vail. The center was founded by Dr. Richard Steadman in 1988 and employs the country's leading orthopedic and sports medicine physicians. My physician specializes in disorders of the hand, wrist, and elbow; and he has special interests in trauma, arthroscopy, and sports-related disorders of the wrist, forearm, and elbow.

I was in superior hands. However, when my orthopedic doctor told me it was the worst wrist injury he had seen and operated on in years, I began to understand the severity of my injuries. It was at that moment I had to make a decision to eliminate fear and be brave. I was in the hospital for five days in which time I had two surgeries. In order to keep the swelling down, I had my arm iced constantly and pain pills were recommended, which I took only when the pain became unbearable. I went home with a huge bandage wrapping and the external fixator to hold my bones in place. There was a two-week break before I re-entered the hospital to have my third surgery.

This time, I had to remain in the hospital for a week. The tissue swelling prevented my doctor from closing up the wound site. Before one of my surgeries, the pre-op medical assistant turned on the Wimbledon tennis match for me to watch while I waited to go into surgery. I tried to make my days there as pleasant and least stressful as possible. After three attempts the doctor succeeded. During that stay I was permitted to walk around and even go to therapy. It was the Fourth of July and I got permission to watch the parade outside. I asked to have my supplements brought to me because I wanted to continue my vitamin routine. My daughters brought me healthy food to eat. I chatted with the staff as I wandered through the hallways. My room was on the same floor where several of my grandchildren had been born.

On the day I emerged from the hospital, I felt a profound sense of gratitude and freedom. I smelled the fresh summer air and lifted my head toward the radiant sun. I was free at last. The last of my stitches came out after 7 weeks while the titanium external fixator remained attached to my arm. My younger grandchildren looked in wonderment at the titanium apparatus and asked if it hurt. I told them "no" and that their Nonna was an 'iron woman." My doctor said I was "braver than a bear." I imagine he was referring to a grizzly.

My hand therapy was twice a week at a Sports Medicine Center in Colorado which specializes in orthopedics and sports medicine; the therapists provide rehabilitative therapies for many of the world's most prominent business and government leaders, elite athletes, and celebrated entertainers. Then there is me, a single active woman in her upper 60's who has prided herself on never breaking a bone in her life —until now. Each session I would ask my therapist more questions and she provided deeper insight into helping me through this arduous healing cycle. I looked forward to my PT sessions for the last year because it gave me much more mobility than I might have had without the therapy.

Initially, I was given the "six pack" exercises which help to move my fingers and stretch my tendons, making me feel as stiff as an arthritic person at times. I learned how to wrap each finger to help stretch my fingers, applying special creams for the scars. I purchased a paraffin machine in order to dip my hand into the hot wax to help with healing. When I looked back, it seemed surreal, and looking forward seemed hopeful. My bones healed up and I gained back more motion and strength. The next part was to have the external hardware removed. This was an immense relief for me after wearing it for two months. Titanium is a light metal but lugging it around felt like lead. I had to sleep with my right arm extended because of the fixator being attached. I couldn't bathe without a rubber sleeve to keep the arm from becoming infected. I still went to the fitness center and managed to do the stationary bike. Then, eleven months after my fall, three titanium plates were removed.

Rather than giving up, I confirmed to myself that I'm a strong woman with a deep belief in healing. I have taken bone density supplements, undergone acupuncture treatments and slowly regained my physical strength with weights, cardio, Pilates and yoga classes. I have been extremely dedicated in gaining back my strength and flexibility. My other arm compensated for my injury and often would go numb especially when I was asleep. My injured arm had lost its muscle strength and the tendons ached constantly. After a year of therapy, I had turned a corner in my healing process. I had to live in each moment and convince myself that I could get through these challenges. I refused to re-live the accident in my mind knowing it would not serve me any purpose; rather I concentrated on balancing my days with rest, exercise, laughter, nutrition and serenity.

My medical bills are another story. I had to give the hospital in Nassau almost $3,000 just to be an outpatient for one day before I left for Colorado. I had no insurance coverage for that—it never crossed my mind that I could injure myself while traveling. I am now looking into travelers insurance for the future. Back in the U.S., I have Medicare, which covers 80% of the bills. I realized I needed to get supplemental insurance, but it went into effect after my surgeries. So my bills are high. I have gone from being debt free to perhaps facing more bills. My life was turned upside down in a matter of minutes.

I have immense gratitude for my family and friends, doctors, nurses and therapists who came to my rescue. My belief in healing one step at a time and receiving encouragement from family and the medical community made my road smoother. As I reflect back on that day, I count my blessings. I could have hit my head or broken my hip or leg. Miracles do happen if you believe.

The time to adopt a healthier lifestyle is always now. Physical activity balanced with a sharp mind and a peaceful nature, plus nutritious food, loving people, and arts and music surrounding you—these are the secrets to being the most vibrant and joyful person you can be, whether you are 50, 60, or 100. My desire and my prayer are to communicate this knowledge to you in a way that sparks your entire being and feeds your soul.

Mind, Attitude and Health: The Benefits

"Mind is the master power that moulds and makes,
And man is mind, and evermore he takes
The tool of thought, and shaping what he wills,
Brings forth a thousand joys, a thousand ills."

~ JAMES ALLEN

While researching information for this book, I was reminded that a healthy life includes how our mind perceives things and how we react to the world around us. It's about eating healthy foods, surrounding ourselves with good friends and a nurturing family. Of course, we don't have control over other people's actions—unless their actions are causing us physical or mental harm. So, controlling the world around us means controlling our inner world. So how can we do this?

One important discovery I've made along the line is to get to know my true self. What does this mean? I am not easily influenced by what I hear from others or read in the newspaper or watch on television. When I was injured I heard some people say "so debilitating" and "it's going to take you a long time to recover," but I refused to be influenced by someone else's opinion of me and my current situation. It is vital for me to seek my own truths in order for me to become my true self.

If we are faced with an illness or an accident, how do we choose to address it? Suppose we have been told we have cancer and the only way to fight it is through chemotherapy, radiation, and drugs. That is precisely what my sister was told by her doctor. She tried to cure herself in Africa by taking a native brew. She went to Cuban women in Florida who prepared herbs for her. When none of this helped she took the traditional route as the doctors prescribed. She informed me that if she didn't do this she would die. During treatment, she became violently sick and weak. The cancer spread, and she died several months later. My sister never believed she would get well. She became desperate and refused to stop working until the day her strength gave out. Fear took over her life.

In my own life and since my accident, I have realized that my mind may have played an even larger part than I realized in my overall health and healing. I had a compound fracture, and was in another country being treated. My doctor in Colorado had concerns that I could develop a bone disease from the fall, especially because it was exposed, and if the immediate medical treatment in Nassau wasn't performed properly. I refused to imagine that would be happening to me. So while flying home which was a very long trip, I prayed and sent positive energy to my injury which gave me calmness and peace. My tolerance for pain increased, and I was more capable of handling my situation with less stress and a clearer mind.

Creating Positive Attitudes Along with Healthy Habits can Make us Truly Happier People

"Happiness is 50% genetic, and the rest is up to us," says David Lykken, a University of Minnesota researcher. To many, happiness doesn't come from being rich and prosperous or owning 'things'. Take in life's small pleasures, make an effort to stay healthy, and focus your energy inward instead of outward. Create and sustain meaningful relationships with family and friends. Consider engaging in a worthwhile philanthropic endeavor or connecting with your church.

Author Gregg Easterbrook writes, "Research shows that people who are grateful, optimistic and forgiving have better experiences with their lives; more happiness, fewer strokes, and higher incomes. If you are looking for something to complain about, you are absolutely certain to find it. It requires some effort to achieve a happy outlook on life and most people don't make it. Most people take the path of least resistance. Far too many people today don't make the steps to make their life more fulfilling."

Heart disease is the number one killer in the United States, accounting for more than 40% of all deaths annually. A study done by the National Institute of Aging involved 229 Chicago-area men and women, ages 50 to 68. It showed that people who say they are lonely have higher blood pressure, which contributes to heart disease. Their systolic blood pressure was 10 to 30 points higher than average. Harvard and Duke Universities found a similar result in people who isolated themselves. Based on these findings, it appears that not only do we need other people for survival; we need them for longevity and well-being. I live alone and yet I am not lonely. I surround myself with a supportive and loving network of family and friends. I participate in activities that include other like-minded individuals.

Doctors have long acknowledged the influence our thought patterns have on the body, but usually only among themselves. Freshman medical texts sometimes admit that as much as 50% of disease is psychosomatic; in other words, "of the mind." Many physicians may fear admitting that much of disease rooted in the mind would put them out of business, leaving only psychiatrists to practice medicine.

Recently, however, we are hearing a few forthright M.D.s actually speaking publicly about the effect of one's thoughts upon the physical body. Take, for instance, the placebo effect. According to a French psychiatrist, Patrick Lemoine, almost 40% of pills prescribed by doctors are 'impure' meaning that they only contain a small amount of medicine in a sugar pill which doesn't medically assist the patient in getting better. Yet the doctor prescribes the pill, and the patient's mind believes there will be an improvement. There are many cases of placebo effects on patients with heart disease as well as Parkinson's. Another more extreme case of mind over matter is the remarkable story of a Spanish doctor, Angel Escudero, who has performed over 900 surgeries without anesthesia. Dr. Escudero performed surgery on a woman who had a severe leg deformity. By making sure her mouth was lubricated with her own saliva and telling herself she was anesthetized, her brain relaxed and the pain receptors were turned off.

In China, medical doctors have long applied acupuncture, a two-thousand-year-old method of inserting needles in various parts of the body. In 1958 acupuncture was used to block pain receptors during surgery to remove tonsils.

Mao Tse Tung, the Chinese leader, mandated that all medical procedures were to be done using acupuncture rather than anesthesia. Acupuncture can divert feelings of pain; however other sensations may be felt. Today, the Chinese doctors use acupuncture primarily on head and neck surgeries.

The eloquent and increasingly popular Dr. Deepak Chopra tells how an individual thought can instantly impact the body via the creation of a neurotransmitter or hormone. Norman Cousins, author of "Anatomy of an Illness," was diagnosed in 1964 with Ankylosing Spondylitis (crippling collagen disease). His doctor gave him a one in 500 chance of recovery. After a series of standard hospital procedures, Cousins checked himself out of the hospital and moved into a hotel. He believed that positive attitudes would result in positive results. Surrounding himself with funny movies and alternative healing methods such as intravenous Vitamin C therapy, he made a full recovery. After reading Dr. Cousin's story, I thought back to my mother. How much did emotions play a part in her theumatoid arthritis (RA), immune system, and health? During the 1960's, psychiatrist George Salomon was an early pioneer in psychoneuroimmunology (PNI), the study of mind/ body connection. He observed the connection between depression and people with RA noting that their depression seemed to make their condition worse.

Dr. David Felton, neurobiologist of the University of Rochester School of Medicine and expert in the field of FNI, has made a remarkable discovery linking the immune system and central nervous system together—all of which is controlled by the brain. A network of nerves from our brain sends signals to the cells of the immune system producing the body/mind connection. Attitudes, feelings, and emotions can have a direct bearing on the immune system.

An Arizona physician, Robert Koppen, M.D., has written: "Thought, combined with feeling, generates a strong creative energy that will not fail to bring about results in the physical world; and whether or not the one who has these thoughts and feelings believes this to be true makes no difference." Dr. Koppen goes on to say that "the bodies and mind connection is a two-edged sword. If we are in a happy, contented, peaceful state of mind, and appreciate the beauty of nature as an expression of Divine intelligence and love, then our thoughts and feelings will amplify the beauty of our world and the health of our body that can be enjoyed. But if we are unhappy, angry, blaming the world, ourselves or God for our self-generated and perpetuated misery, then the physical results of our inner attitude can become quite destructive to our mental, emotional and physical health."

> *"Your living is determined not so much by what life brings to you as by the attitude you bring to life; not so much by what happens to you as by the way your mind looks at what happens."*
>
> - KAHLIL GIBRAN

A Stroke's Silver Lining

In 1996, at age 37, Dr. Jill Bolte Taylor, a Harvard-trained neuroanatomist, suffered a severe stroke. Upon waking one morning, she felt disoriented and began to notice a sensitivity to sound and body sensations, among other symptoms. While showering, she noticed her hands appeared to look like claws, her body was rigid and the slightest noises became extreme to her. It took Dr. Taylor about 4 hours to recognize she had had a stroke that affected the left hemisphere of her brain. When her right arm became paralyzed; she knew for sure it was a major stroke. Going into her home office, she tried to recognize her office number on her business card, but her reasoning and language skills were not there. When she finally managed to call her office, she was unable to form words. Fortunately, her associate answered the phone, recognized her voice and, knowing something was not right, called 911. Upon entering Massachusetts General Hospital, Dr. Taylor had no understanding of whom the people were who asked her to sign some papers. During her hospital stay the medical staff appeared distant and unconcerned about her or her condition. A woman she knew in the professional field whom she dubbed "The Queen of Neurology," entered her room with an entourage of medical students. Dr. Taylor felt safe around this person because she sensed familiarity and respect coming from her, though she did not know her. When her mother, Gigi, arrived, Dr. Taylor had no idea who she was, or for that matter, what a mother was. Gigi crawled into bed with her daughter and held her.

> *"All I knew was this loving, kind, spirit came in, wrapped herself around me and just took ownership of loving me—and that was the new beginning"*
>
> ~ DR. JILL BOLTE TAYLOR "MY STROKE OF INSIGHT"

After 5 days, Dr. Taylor went home where her mother took care of her. Two and a half weeks later, she underwent surgery to remove a tumor from the left hemisphere of her brain. It took 8 years for her to completely recover from the stroke. She had to re-learn language and left-brain activities, which had virtually disappeared from her memory. Dr. Taylor says it was like a re-birth. On the one hand, her right brain which holds the feelings, intuitive, and creative parts was amped up. Disconnected from ego and reasoning, she felt this incredible presence of peace and joy, even though she couldn't speak or understand what was going on around her. On the other hand, her right brain was demonstrating a state of peace and nirvana.

Today, Dr. Taylor has an 'attitude of gratitude' and is able to filter out thoughts from her left brain that do not contribute to her mental health and wholeness. While her long recovery was clearly difficult, in the process she came to believe that we as a species are 99% identical, thus making us interconnected beings. Essentially, she realized there is really no separation between us. The left brain has the ability to analyze, feel a sense of ego, reason, use vocabulary, and identify functions. Dr. Taylor says that through this life-altering experience, she has been capable of altering the circuitry that runs through her brain cells, whether conscious or subconscious, to create new rules.

Dr. Taylor is passionately involved as a national spokesperson for the mentally ill and supports postmortem studies on people with schizophrenia and bipolar disorders. She also lends her talent as a musician and travels the country as the Singing Scientist. In 2009, Time Magazine awarded Dr. Taylor one of the 100 Most Influential People in the World. She has also been featured on Oprah's Soul Series web cast as well as in interviews with Dr. Oz and Oprah Winfrey.

After listening to Dr. Taylor's story, I have a greater understanding and compassion for my mother, who I'm fairly certain had the ability to observe, but not to communicate. When my mother suffered a stroke at 53, I was living in Florida. I remember trying to comprehend what she was saying to me over the phone as her stroke had impaired her speech. This made her difficult to understand. I could sense her fear and how distraught she sounded, so I kept telling her I loved her and would travel up north to be with her. Sadly, while I was on the trip there, my mother died. How difficult it must have been for her to want to be understood, but not be able to speak clearly to me. My mother always had a controlling personality, and this time she was not able to control what was happening to her body or her mind.

"All that we are is the result of what we have thought. If a man speaks or acts with an evil thought, pain follows him. If a man

speaks or acts with a pure thought, happiness follows him, like a shadow that never leaves him."

— BUDDHA

Mind Over Matter

Several years ago I was asked to donate time to help a group of young people prepare for a Special Olympics swim meet. I felt that I was in a sea of carefree adults in a childlike mind who were so enthusiastic about achieving their goal of swimming from one end of the pool to the other. I was able to communicate with them by getting close, focusing on their faces, and praising them. After our practice sessions, we took the group to the indoor hot tub where they could get warm before heading to the locker room to shower and change. One day, while entering the tubs, another small group of adults seemed to become very uncomfortable with our group, and immediately got out of the pool. Even though it didn't seem to impact our group, it seemed similar to the cold manner of the hospital staff tending to Dr. Taylor. When we treat one another with open respect, kindness and caring, we all benefit.

In the late 1990's, I was living in a small mountain community in the southwest corner of Colorado. I visited with a German scientist, Adolph Zielinski, who had come to town to try to help a friend of mine who was suffering from a brain tumor. Dr. Zielinski had worked closely with several Russian scientists to decipher and study the brain, much like Dr. Taylor, before and after her stroke. He had traveled around the world using certain right and left brain techniques to help stimulate the deeper realms of the brain and activate four stages of brain waves: Beta (waking stage), alpha (meditative, day dreaming), theta (creativity, dreams), delta (deep sleep, out of body experiences). During his stay, I was introduced to the various brain waves through a series of sounds of various frequencies that I listened to with a headset. The session lasted an hour. I believe that the frequencies heightened the portion of my brain that stimulated the taste buds. One of the first things I noticed afterwards was how food tasted to me. It was as though I had never experienced these tastes before, and they were wonderful. All my senses seemed to be heightened, and a feeling of euphoria surrounded me. I could still think and reason, but my left side of the brain seemed less in command.

A few days after Dr. Zelinski left, I awoke one morning feeling different in my head. I saw rapid pictures as though I was watching a movie in fast forward. I thought, "How strange," and began to feel that the brain-wave session was producing some differences in my brain. I was wondering if I could drive to my office. Everything else seemed normal so I decided it was safe for me to operate my vehicle. Once at my office, I realized my focus and my left brain activities weren't stimulated. The fast-forward images had continued. I left the office and stayed home for two days observing this phenomenon and having a joyful time. On the third day, when I awoke, something was different. The images had faded, my euphoria had diminished, and I felt once again like my original self. It made me sad—I wished I could have maintained the feelings that had given me such a beautiful experience.

Perhaps we can achieve a visceral experience each day of our lives by applying various principles in our own lives, including integrating gratitude and wholeness toward ourselves and others by recognizing that we are all powerful inter-connected beings that truly wish to be appreciated and loved.

Scientific Findings

In Bruce Lipton's book," The Biology of Belief," scientific findings merge with a convergence of the body-mind-spirit trinity to empower our thoughts, beliefs and attitudes into our daily lives. We are living in a world filled with chaotic energy which affects our path to peace-filled living. Bruce Lipton's scientific studies have shown that our childhood beliefs and programmed perceptions can be radically shifted and help to rewrite our genetic coding. His research is in tune with "The Power of Positive Thinking" and "The Laws of Attraction." His new science of cellular biology can inspire us personally and professionally.

> *"I have learned to think of everything I see as having an energetic template that makes it appear as it does in the physical. When I want to change something in my life, I start with changing my energy. I do that by changing my belief about it and the emotions that I associate with it. It might sound crazy, but that is what the Law of Attraction is all about."*
>
> - Bruce Lipton Ph.D.

The mind-bending movie "Groundhog Day" concerns a reporter who is on assignment in Punxsutawney, Pennsylvania to televise whether or not the groundhog will see his shadow, indicating six more weeks of winter. This self-centered man hates this reporting assignment, and has lived by controlling his life every day of his existence. What occurs in the film is that he continues to repeat the same day which begins in his hotel room with the radio playing Sonny and Cher's "I Got You Babe." One morning he has an epiphany of how much he has suffered in life by trying to control his existence. He then realizes how miserable he is because of his continual attachment to his desires. Somewhere in the middle of this poignant story, he knows there is a way out of suffering through doing good deeds, through right thought, right action, right speech and right living. He becomes liberated and joyful. In the end, he finds his true love, happiness in living life outside of his selfish interests, and he no longer has to repeat the same day over and over. He creates a new day in Punxsutawney. As the singer Jimi Hendrix once said "The power of love overcomes the love of power."

De-stress, Naturally

Cortisol and Stress

Do you have any of the following health challenges: Type 1 and 2 diabetes, muscle loss, heart disease, memory loss, depression, high blood pressure, obesity or autoimmune disease? If so, the stress hormone, cortisol, may be affecting your health.

When we're stressed, suffer physical trauma or extreme physical exertion, our cortisol level increases to help maintain homeostasis. However, our cortisol levels also increase as we age and may stay high for longer periods of time, which can be extremely toxic. Brain cells are sensitive to the effects of cortisol; excess cortisol could cause damage to the brain cells, compromise the immune system, decrease muscle mass and shrink organs.

When we suffer from unmanaged stress, our thyroid glands are impaired and adrenals go into overload. I personally have an acute sense of adrenal burnout, and experience symptoms such as extreme agitation. When this happens, I take stock of my emotions and activities, rest more, and am determined to have more fun and relaxation in my life. I also watch what I eat and drink, monitor my thoughts, and remove myself from any stressful and disruptive outside disturbances.

De-stress and release dis-ease

Stress is closely linked to many diseases. Studies have shown that stress causes immune systems to become compromised and produce higher levels of interleukin-6, a protein that modulates immune responses. When IL-6 measures in higher concentrations, it can accelerate colds, flu and other illnesses, as well as contribute to poorer cognitive functioning. Plasma fibrinogen in the bloodstream indicates the presence of inflammation. When we are under stress, we produce higher levels of this chemical, which may compromise heart health. Happy people produce lower levels of plasma fibrinogen. This is another reason to smile.

In the past decade, a worldwide increase in depression has lead to a rise in the use of anti-depressants globally. By the year 2020, depression may be considered the number 2 cause of disease worldwide, according to the World Health Organization. Would you care to venture a guess as to how many people are on anti-depressants in the United States? Try 18.8 million.

Prozac, Zoloft and Paxil are just a few anti-depressants in the market place. A couple members of my family have taken them at one time or another. I understand they can be useful for some people. My choice so far is to seek other ways to achieve peace and happiness without a doctor's prescription. If you are considering or have been taking anti-depressants, ask your pharmacist and doctor what kind of side effects there may be. Education is your best resource.

Mind-Enhancing Transmitters

Depression has a lot to do with nutrition and mood transmitters. For instance, if we lack energy mentally and physically, we may turn to coffee or sugar as temporary stimulants. Instead of coffee or sugar, one may consider 5-Hydroxytryptophan (5-HTP), an amino acid which enhances serotonin levels in the brain. Another option is L-Tryptophan, an amino acid that also is a neurotransmitter for our brain, taken before bed. In only one month, you may notice a shift in your feelings—all for the better. You may feel more positive, easy-going, and better able to handle stress.

L-Tryptophan is found in high-protein foods such as turkey, pork, beef, chicken, eggs, and dairy products. Many vegetarians produce lower-than-normal levels of serotonin, so in these cases supplementing with L-Tryptophan can be a good idea. Consult with your practitioner before taking supplements.

Endorphins

The body produces three categories of endorphins: beta (usually released in the pituitary gland), enkephalins and dynorphins, which are associated with the nervous system. Some food sources that produce endorphins include chocolate and spicy chili peppers. Endorphins reduce pain in the body, act as an appetite modulator, release sex hormones, and create feelings of euphoria like "runner's high." Endorphins also enhance the immune system and help delay the aging process. Furthermore, they can play a crucial role in helping drug and alcohol abusers overcome their addictions. When our endorphins are low, we may avoid intimacy or confrontation, handle our emotions in an unhealthy manner, and/or turn to substances such as drugs, alcohol, and food. Stimulating the production of endorphins through exercise can help the addictions to subside.

Endorphins are naturally produced by a wide range of activities like hearty laughter, meditation and/or deep breathing, acupuncture or chiropractic treatments. Tyrosine is an amino acid that helps increase the production of endorphins in the body. It's considered a natural antidepressant, assisting in producing thyroid hormones, which is a basic factor in our adrenals. Tyrosine is considered one of our most pleasure-promoting chemicals. The molecular structure of Tyrosine is very similar to morphine but with different chemical properties. Tyrosine, which is produced in the body from phenylalanine, is found in soy products, chicken, turkey, fish, peanuts, almonds, avocados, bananas, milk, cheese, yogurt, cottage cheese, lima beans, pumpkin seeds, and sesame seeds.

Phenylalanine is also very similar to tyrosine in that it produces euphoria and helps subdue pain. D-phenylalanine is a very potent endorphin. GABA (gamma amino butyric acid) is both an amino acid and a neurotransmitter. GABA helps alleviate stress and acts as a natural Valium.

Brain Food from the Sea

In a current study at Rush University Medical Center in Chicago, Dr.

Martha Clare Morris has followed 3,718 people 65 and older for 6 years. Participants ate fish high in omega-3 fatty acids, which included DHA (Docosahexaenoic acid), which is responsible for early brain development. Those over 65 who ate fish twice or more a week showed their rate of cognitive decline reduced 10 to 13% per year. Eating deep-sea fish like salmon, cod or halibut at least once a week reduced their mental aging by as much as 3 years.

Nutrition ~ Exercise and Sleep for Our Brain

Diet, exercise and sleep are vital components in reducing brain aging. Nutrition plays an important role in keeping our brain smart. Breakfast that supplies protein, not sugar, gives the brain a jumpstart. Eggs are rich in acetylcholine, a neurotransmitter. Low levels of this have been linked to patients with Alzheimer's. Salads are packed with antioxidants to help prevent free radicals from forming and provide better cognitive skills. Yogurt contains tyrosine, an amino acid, which helps our memory and alertness. Fruits, in particular blueberries and strawberries, help improve our memory, coordination and concentration. Eating healthy foods promotes our overall well being.

Exercising boosts our cognitive abilities. It may be as simple as taking a walk several times a week. Our brain can grow new cells, and exercising helps achieve this. Yoga has many different movements which are forward and backwards. Backward bends seem to boost the mental state, which could explain why I feel elated after class. A good night's sleep recharges our brain cells. There may be moments during our sleep in which we can create new thought and wake up with creative new ideas in our head. In this section there is more description on the benefits of a good night's sleep.

Brain Injuries

Could there be a link between people who suffer brain damage from blood hemorrhages, automobile accidents and falls? Dr. Sandra Magnoni of the Ospedale Maggiore Policlinico Trauma Center in Milan, Italy inserted a catheter into 18 patients' brains for 3 to 7 days to observe the beta-amyloid level (an Alzheimer's-related protein). The Amyloid-beta measurements may indicate how well the cells are communicating with each other. In Alzheimer's patients, a sticky gooey form rather than a fluid bathes the brain. Scientists have not yet connected the purpose of the Beta-amyloid or what triggers the plaque formations within the brain. A person with brain injuries may develop dementia later in life. If continued studies and research can show a link between brain damage and increased Beta-amyloid connection, it may help to lower the risk of Alzheimer's disease

Preventing Alzheimer's

Today, 5.1 million people in the United States suffer from Alzheimer's disease. It is the seventh leading cause of death and affects one in eight people age 65 and older and one-half of those 85 and older. More than 26 million people worldwide were estimated to be living with Alzheimer's disease in 2006, according to a study led by researchers at the Johns Hopkins Bloomberg School of Public Health. This figure could grow to 106 million by 2050. In Asia, over 48% of Alzheimer cases are currently documented.

Dr Gary Small Study

The University of California, along with Dr. Gary Small, performed a 14-day study of 34 adults with average memories and an average age of 53 years. They were asked to perform a series of functions, including behavior modification, brisk walks and physical conditioning, along with stretching and relaxation techniques. They were also put on a memory improvement plan that included exercises such as crossword puzzles and brain teasers. They ate 5 small meals per day featuring Omega-3 fats from fish and olive oil, whole grain carbohydrates, and antioxidants.

At the beginning and end of the 14-day trial, the volunteers were given a PET (positron emission tomography) scan that measured activity throughout the brain. Results showed that memory improved while using less brain power. Dr. Small states that "it is never too late or too early to get started on a healthy lifestyle to improve your brain power."

Another study by the MacArthur Foundation found that seniors who were physically active maintained a higher level of brain function over a 10-year period dating from the beginning of the study. Also, genetics don't always play a dominant role mentally and physically; regular exercise can outweigh the genetic blueprint.

Hope for Alzheimer's

It appears that the longer one lives, the higher the risk of developing Alzheimer's. The disease has been linked to a protein known as beta-amyloid, which collects between nerve cells, thus disrupting brain function and triggering an immune response that destroys the cells. Scientists have been testing viable new drugs, which will give hope to those with low to moderate levels of the disease.

Sam Gandy, chairman of the National Medical and Scientific Advisory Council of the Alzheimer's Association and Director of the Farber Institute for Neurosciences in Philadelphia, presented the following statement to the Aging Subcommittee, Senate Health, Education, and Labor and Pensions Committee in March 2007.

"Within 3 years, it's all but certain we'll have disease-modifying drugs that fundamentally change the nature of Alzheimer's," he said.

A United States research study has shown that people who take angiotension-receptor blockers are 35 to 40% less likely to develop Alzheimer's disease. Angiotension-receptor blockers are drugs that are used to lower blood pressure. In addition to the good news with respect to preventing Alzheimer's disease, the study showed that even if a person already has the illness, starting the angiotension-receptor blockers would slow the progression of the illness down by 45%. Professor Clive Ballard of the Alzheimer's Research Society is quoted as saying, "This study highlights that it is becoming increasingly important to investigate blood-pressure lowering drugs as a potential treatment for dementia."

A new report became available in 2010 which is an analysis of existing therapeutics available for AD.

How to Join a Clinical Trial

When it comes to Alzheimer's, buying any time at all is a good idea. Therefore early detection is a key to slowing the disease, and researchers urge participation in clinical trials. "To take part in a trial is a great gift to society," says William Thies, Vice President of Medical and Scientific Relations for the Alzheimer's Association.

To find out about clinical trials and studies in your area refer to the reference section at the back of this book.

A Daughter's Approach to Alzheimer Disease

My friend Sally traveled to Vermont to visit her parents who are in their 90s. Her dad lived at home and her mom had been in a care facility for the last 3 years because it became increasingly difficult for her dad to watch over her, though he traveled a few short miles each day to visit and have dinner with her. When my friend was there, she asked her mom (who does not recognize her daughter anymore) if she would like to let her husband know she is tired and wishes to leave her body. Sally said her mom's face lit up and she nodded. So Sally took the big step in talking to her dad about this incident. Her father went to see her mother, but would not discuss any of the sharing that Sally and her mom had.

Sally feels that if her dad would tell her mother that it is OK for her to leave her body, she would. Sally feels her dad is holding on to his wife emotionally, and that she senses this. Her condition continues to deteriorate, and she rarely goes outside. Sally realizes that she needs to leave this heartbreaking situation in the hands of her father. Recently her father's deteriorating health led to the decision for her father to move into the same facility that his wife is in. He has major diabetes and had heart bypass surgery 10 years ago. Sally's mother has moved from the Alzheimer's floor to the general ailment section of the care facility. Now they spend days together eating meals and seeing each other. Sally's dad has learned to accept help easier since he doesn't live in his own home or drive his car any longer.

Sally's loving story reminds me of Nicholas Spark's book, *The Notebook,* in which two people married and lived devotedly for many years. The wife developed Alzheimer's and didn't recognize her family or husband except for brief moments. Her husband moved into the same facility where they passed away serenely in each other's arms. There are various stories which contain different dynamics around family members who have Alzheimer's.

How do we care for our loved ones and how can we afford to have them in an extended care facility? Can we care for them in their home or have them move into ours? The Alzheimer's Foundation of America is an excellent resource to help guide people through the process and help create a better quality of life.

Cultivating a Healthy Mind and Brain

I offer the following suggestions as catalysts for your continuing quest for improved immunity and vitality.

I. Be grateful: Develop an "Attitude of Gratitude."

When there is something that may not be going well, rather than focusing on what is wrong and how you can fix it, ask yourself "what do I have in my life right now to be grateful for?" This simple exercise doesn't make problems go away but rather makes them less important for the moment. Focusing on gratitude can help you can find a solution to the current situation, as you are better able to cope with difficulties by addressing them with a gracious and grateful nature.

• Rather than concentrating on what you don't have, give thanks for each day by focusing on the amazing things in your life
• Make a list of people and things in your life you are grateful for
• Greet people with a smile or do something kind for another
• Don't allow pressures in your life to let you forget to be grateful

II. Be Creative- Express Yourself in Artful Ways

We are never too old to create. It could be painting a sunset, throwing a piece of pottery on the wheel, touring an art museum, looking at beautiful architecture or just allowing your imagination to run wild. Remember as children we eagerly dove into finger painting, coloring, drawing or making clay objects. I have taken classes in both stained glass and weaving; they were challenging as well as extremely rewarding. I have also studied pottery and look forward to making a clay piece some day soon. Recently I have been taking my camera with me to capture various images—creative activities, all.

• Boost your intuitive nature by taking an art class
• Read books
• Write a story
• Visit an art museum or exhibit
• Take photographs of images that inspire you
• Create a beautiful space in your home or garden

III. Be Active- Get Out and Move

An active body keeps our minds sharp and creates more flexibility in our lives. Sitting around too much drags us down and compromises our health. You don't have to become a professional athlete. I weave in and out of yoga and Pilates classes. Each day I do something to keep my heart pumping and my body strong knowing that I am taking care of myself through exercise and a healthy diet.

- Take walks or bike whenever you can and leave your car at home
- Join a Pilates, yoga or weight training class and have fun
- Strive to do things that you thought you could not do
- Stretch your body and breathe deeply during the day
- Take up an outdoor sport—learn how to ski, swim or even sail

IV. Be Inspired

Inspiration means to be 'in spirit' and comes from being fully present and full of vitality each day. We may be inspired by looking at the starlit night or hearing a beautiful symphony. Often when I am working on a book project I let my imagination take hold. I may read a passage that inspires or witness a wondrous sunset; listen to beautiful music or go for a swim. Inspiration keeps us bursting open and makes us feel more alive. It is an internal feeling that touches each of us in unique ways. Live expressively by filling your home with flowers, music, and anything that inspires you. Accept and expect all that is good in life, both inside and out, and discover your unique role in life—what brings you passion and enthusiasm?

- Read inspiring books
- Leap into action by doing something worthwhile for your community or an organization
- Turn off the television, radio, and other distractions and sit quietly and listen to that still voice within
- Inspire others by sharing your own purpose through ideas and abilities
- Be true to yourself and your ideals

V. Connect With Nature

As a child I relished living outdoors in the summertime. I would canoe miles of lakes or river inlets hearing the bottom of my boat go 'swoosh' over the water lilies while observing the ambitious beavers piling wood to build their homes. I swam every day, sometimes for miles across the lake or went hiking on a trail or up a mountain. Sometimes I found myself simply lying in a field of wild flowers while the honey bees drank nectar. One period of my life I volunteered at the Audubon Preserve along the shores of Lake Michigan. Nature has always given me peace of mind and a great appreciation for life.

• Get out in nature and witness the natural beauty and stillness around you
• Live around nature if at all possible
• If you live in the city, visit a park or arboretum
• Sign up for nature hikes and programs
• Listen to the sounds of nature

> *"Climb the mountains and get their good tidings. Nature's peace will flow into you as sunshine flows into trees. The winds will blow their own freshness into you, and the storms their energy, while cares will drop off like autumn leaves."*
>
> - John Muir[1]

VI. Be Selfish - Treat - Pamper Yourself

Being selfish is a difficult thing for many of us to aspire to. And yet it is important for us to learn how to be kinder to ourselves. I raised 5 children, and had very little time to do things for myself that didn't involve the family. I disciplined myself to make time for just me. Sometimes I was able to squeeze an hour away. Sometimes it was as simple as a walk or a lunch with a friend. In the long run it made me a more tolerant and happier mother and wife. Serve yourself. You deserve it.

• Schedule a day at a spa for a massage and facial
• Have lunch with a friend
• Have your family do the chores for a day
• See a play or listen to a concert
• Soak in a long bath and don't forget to lock the door

VII. Be Mellow

Let's face it. We live in a complicated and stressful world. You may live in a big city and commute to work or you may currently be out of work. There may be an illness or other challenge within your family. You may live alone and find your life lonely and uninspiring. There are ways to counter stress; each person copes with stress in their own way. You may internalize it and keep it bottled up inside. You may become extremely agitated and angry. You may drink, eat unhealthy foods, take drugs or smoke too much. You may get panic attacks or make yourself ill. The cortisol level in our body increases as we age, affecting our brain cells and immune system. Stress also creates higher levels of cortisol, which helps to create the stubborn fat in the stomach that we can't seem to lose no matter what we do. There are ways to counter stress with the following suggestions.

- Herbs (check with your practitioner if on a prescribed medicine); Serenity® by Gaia Herbs, usually found in a health store or online, contains Kava Kava and other herbs to steady the nerves
- Refer to supplement section which addresses ways you can alleviate stress, including Tyrosine, Phenylalanine and GABA

Benefits of Meditation

- Meditation increases the thickness of the cerebral cortex—an area of the brain associated with sensory and attention processes.
- Meditation can bring calmness, peace and a joyful expression
- Meditation can help reduce stress and pain
- Helps with respiratory and cardiovascular functions
- Reduces stress, improves the immune system and lowers blood pressure

Take supplements: Tyrosine, Phenylalanine and GABA which helps to alleviate stress.

Learn breathing techniques. Close your eyes - breathe normally through your nose—be aware of breathing in and out. Expand belly as you inhale, belly in as you exhale. Do count of 4 for each in and out.

Author meditating in her thirties

VIII. Be Rested - How to have a Good Night's Sleep

My 75-year-old grandmother who had Diabetes Mellitus Type 2 would often read a book in the middle of the night. One time I asked her why. Her response was simply "At my age, I can't afford to sleep." I understood her intentions and yet, a good night's sleep is important for our well being. Dr. Eve Van Cauter at the University of Chicago found that chronic sleep deprivation—defined as 6.5 hours or less of sleep per night—has the same effect on insulin resistance as aging. Along with poor diet, a sedentary lifestyle, aging and chronic stress, lack of sleep is a risk factor for Type 2 Diabetes.

I sleep 8 to 9 hours each night, and rise early in the morning. There are times I take a 30 minute 'cat nap' during the middle part of the day, with my kitty, of course. My sister was the opposite. She often stayed up till 1 a.m. and still got up early to go to work.

- Avoid bedtime snacks, particularly grains, sugar, caffeine, liquor, high fat or spicy meals; these will raise blood sugar levels, stimulate digestion and make sleep difficult; later, when blood sugar levels drop too low (hypoglycemia), you might wake up and not be able to fall back asleep

- Combining B vitamins with calcium and magnesium can calm your nervous system; beans, turkey, chicken, nuts, eggs, and dairy contain high levels of B vitamins

- Eat foods that enhance serotonin levels (such as salmon, hummus, and baked tempeh) a few hours before bedtime; this helps to balance our sugar levels and provide for a more restful sleep

- Do not watch television or work in bed; read spiritual or inspirational literature for a few minutes before bed, and avoid dramatic novels or distressing reading material; once in bed, close your eyes and simply 'feel' your body—and wherever you notice tension, consciously relax that area—then, simply pay attention to your slow, easy breathing until you fall asleep

- Go to bed as early as possible; prior to the invention of electricity, people went to bed shortly after sundown, as most animals do, which is what nature intended for humans as well. The body systems, particularly the adrenal glands, do a majority of their recovering during the hours of 11 p.m. and 1 a.m. In addition, the gallbladder dumps toxins during this time period; if you are awake, those toxins back up into the liver—which then secondarily back up into your entire system, causing further disruption to your health

- Aim to be in your bed with the lights out between 9:30 and 10:30 p.m.; if you are not used to getting to bed this early, move your bedtime up by thirty minutes every week until you are in bed by 10:30; for example, if you usually watch television until midnight, try turning off the TV at 11:30 for a week; then aim for thirty minutes earlier; and finally to bed at 10:30 p.m.

- Stay away from alcohol; although alcohol makes you drowsy at first, its effect is short-lived and you often wake up after a few hours. Alcohol will also prevent you from falling into the deeper stages of sleep, when the body does most of its healing

- Avoid foods to which you may be sensitive; this is particularly true for dairy and wheat products, because they have been shown to cause sleep apnea, gastrointestinal upset, excess congestion, and gas, among others

- Try to reduce or avoid as many drugs as possible; many medications, both prescription and over-the-counter, may affect sleep.

- Create a peaceful, dark bedroom

- There are a variety of herbs for a sound sleep; some herbal supplement suggestions are Melatonin, Seratonin, Lavender, Chamomile, Hops and Valerian; drink a nighttime herbal tea or soak in an herbal bath

Consult with your practitioner if you are having difficulty sleeping and wish to substitute a more natural approach than prescription medicine.

IV. Be Healthy and Happy

By starting with this book, I hope you have been inspired to become healthier. Being healthy and happy encompasses the food we eat, our daily attitudes, and the environment where we live; which include our community of family and friends. We can choose to change our diet, exercise more or be of service to another who may need help.

I have told Dr. Norman Cousin's story of his illness and his empowering decisions to engage in laughter and heal his medical condition. Anything is possible. Choose happiness each day. It may be as simple as eating a scrumptious juicy apple just picked from a tree. It could be lying in a hammock with one of your grandchildren or witnessing a splendid rainbow after a misty rain. True happiness comes from deep within us.

- Smile every day
- Laugh often
- Eat fresh, healthy foods
- Spend time with family or friends
- Give thanks for your life each day
- Help someone in need

> *"Each morning when I open my eyes I say to myself: I, not events, have the power to make me happy or unhappy today. I can choose which it shall be. Yesterday is dead, tomorrow hasn't arrived yet. I have just one day, today, and I'm going to be happy in it."*
>
> ~ GROUCHO MARX

Be Smart ~ Our Thoughts and Our Choices

Along with peaceful sleep and current mind research, we can be helped with diseases associated with aging. We can also change our mind about life situations. A book and video called *The Secret* made its debut in 2006. It has become a national best-seller and was featured on *The Oprah Winfrey Show*. The gist of the material is the law of attraction, which states that what we believe, we draw into our lives and that becomes our reality. We do not live in a perfect world. But how we react and respond to our earthly experiences molds our identity along with our state of health, peace of mind and consciousness. Who we are evolves from the world we create with our choice of experiences and associations.

If you feel overwhelmed with any situation, put it aside and make a list of all the people and experiences that you are grateful for at this moment in your life. You will see your perspective shift toward a more positive attitude.

> *"Beliefs have the power to create and the power to destroy. Human beings have the awesome ability to take any experience of their lives and create a meaning that disempowers them or one that can literally save their lives."*
>
> ~ ANTHONY ROBBINS

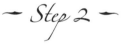

Your Body: The Vehicle That Lasts a Lifetime

How Our Body Image Reflects Wholeness

I have lived my entire life knowing the importance of keeping my body strong, stretched and moving. While my siblings and I were growing up in the 40's and 50's we were as active as any other children. We were rarely inside; we rode our bikes to school, played all kinds of sports and went to summer camp. Even though my grandparents, parents, aunts and uncles were not physically active people (and were not slim, either), my mother had the foresight to send us to camp until we were seventeen, and then my sister and I were tennis instructors at a camp on Lake Champlain, Vermont. My sister had polio before the Salk vaccine came out, so my brother and I were sent away from home until she recovered (her spine gave her difficulty throughout her lifetime). My brother was a football player in high school and college, and being a tall and large muscled person, his weight escalated at times to 260 pounds. He broke his hip in his early 60s while on his bike. It was a painful journey back and to this day one leg is slightly shorter than the other. He recently retired and has high hopes of getting back to an exercise program.

After I married, my family often went camping and my husband and I played doubles in tennis matches. I had horses, skied, hiked, swam and basically continued being physically active. The only time my weight ballooned was when I was in high school. I have had small weight gains through the years but never more than a 10 to 15 pound increase. My sister had an active metabolism so whatever she ate was burned off. As an adult she never prepared meals at home for herself, especially after her divorce. I was flabbergasted when I tried to cook for her when she had cancer. Her dishwasher was never used, her garbage disposal had been broken for two years, and her cooking pots were brand new. She would order takeout food or eat at restaurants. When she was in chemotherapy, I would make her breakfast and we would sit at her dining room table, something she never did. She told me she never ate breakfast at home; instead she would grab a chocolate bar on the way to her office. She worked out at a local gym; however, she seemed off balance when it came to other areas of her life.

Today, skinny models project a perfect Barbie-like figure. At the other end of the spectrum, children and teenagers are becoming more obese, at least in part because schools have eliminated or cut back on gym classes. People sit in front of computer and television screens more frequently, both at home and on the job. 60% of Americans are now classed as overweight. We are flooded with commercials for weight-loss plans and diet pills galore. If we have poor self-esteem it is reflected in drinking, eating, drugs and abusive behavior. The key is to get help and demonstrate a more kind and positive nature toward ourselves. Then we can begin to foster better health *naturally*, through improved foods, exercise, and mental balance.

Exercise and Health: The Benefits

A. Boost Your Metabolism

Our metabolism converts food and stored fat into energy. As we age, our metabolism slows, but exercise can speed it up. Exercise is crucial to a healthy life, especially in our later years.

Basal Metabolic Rate

An important measurement of metabolism is the basal metabolic rate (BMR). The BMR is the amount of energy expended to support basic bodily functions such as your heartbeat, breathing, walking, sleeping, and brain activity. Men typically have a 10 to 15% faster BMR than women. The resting metabolic rate, which is closely related to the BMR, makes up 50 to 75% of our daily caloric expenditure and depends on the size of our bodies.

Research shows that increased daily activity plus a toned physique can help accelerate the body's metabolism. Lean muscle mass makes your metabolism work faster and stronger. Exercising just 30 minutes a day increases muscle mass which helps to keep the metabolic rate higher at any age. Exercise and normal daily activities also aid in burning more calories due to the cells' increased labor. You can also boost your metabolism by eating smaller quantities of food throughout the day rather than three large meals. Avoid trans fats, drink more purified water, and choose whole grain and fresh foods. We'll discuss all of this in detail further in the book.

B. Prevent Joint Pain and Arthritis

My mother had severe rheumatoid arthritis, but not once did her doctors suggest an exercise program for fear that movement would put more stress on her swollen joints. Today, it is known that exercise can help alleviate pain in the knees and hips. Along with more traditional care, current views on the management of arthritis include aerobic exercise and resistance training to strengthen muscles around joints and take the pressure off the joints themselves. Stretching keeps the body flexible, while aerobic exercise can help with weight control, thereby relieving the strain on joints.

C. Osteoporosis

Bone loss can in some cases be reversed and bone health maintained by exercise, including walking and hiking, weight training, stretching and yoga at least 30 minutes to an hour five days a week. You will be rewarded with more flexibility and fewer injuries and falls. Exercise assists in developing muscle strength and building bones. Discuss with your doctor a unique exercise program for your body. If you have developed fractures, consult with your practitioner about the safe way to exercise.

D. Improve Heart Health

We know that regular exercise benefits the cardiovascular system. It strengthens your heart and improves circulation. It in-

Heart Rate

To gain the most from your cardio exercise regimen, first determine your target maximum working heart rate by deducting your age from 220. Once you have that number, during the first few weeks of your exercise program, aim at the lowest part of your target zone (50%). Gradually build up to the higher part of your target zone (75%). After six months of regular exercise, you may be able to exercise comfortably at up to 85% of your maximum heart rate.

creases endurance and lowers blood pressure. It assists in losing unwanted weight. Working at a lower heart rate provides more fat-burning benefits while higher rates provide cardiovascular benefits. Walking, biking, jogging, and swimming are all beneficial exercise. It would be smart to do something every day. If you are an inactive person and have a heart condition, please seek medical advice before beginning any exercise regimen. There are supervised medical athletic centers that provide professional supervision and monitoring during any exercise program. Many of these places are geared toward people who are recovering from heart surgery or have medical conditions that may lead to heart problems.

In my view, machines at health clubs are not that accurate in measuring heart rate. You can purchase a heart-rate monitor on the Internet or through sporting goods or biking stores. It looks like a watch and can be worn anywhere (prices and models vary). A monitor can help you keep track of not only your heart rate, but also your target zone and calories burned.

For example: if you are 50 years old, your target maximum working heart rate would be 170 beats per minute. When you begin your workout regimen, aim for a consistent level of 85 and gradually work up to about 127. When you've maintained this level for six months or more, you may comfortably work up to 144.

D. Lower Cholesterol

There are two types of cholesterol: low-density lipoprotein (LDL) "bad" cholesterol, which can damage the arteries and thus lead to heart disease, and high-density lipoprotein (HDL) which in higher amounts can transport the excess LDL into the liver where it is then transported out of the body. Cholesterol particle size varies. It appears that the larger protein particles are increased during exercise, reducing the harmful smaller particles. Therefore, when we exercise, we lower our "bad" cholesterol count. A study from Duke University Medical Center and East Carolina University tested 111 inactive overweight men and women. People who exercised at least 30 minutes a day were able to lower their LDL rate. The ones who added more vigorous exercise which amounted to up to 20 miles a week of jogging not only lowered LDL but also increased HDL rates. It is possible to jog 20 miles a week on a treadmill, putting in just three miles per day for six to seven days.

E. Diabetes 2 (Adult Onset Diabetes)

In this form of diabetes, the pancreas produces more insulin while sugar builds up in the bloodstream. Genetics, obesity, high LDL levels, smoking, inactive lifestyle and diet play an integral role in whether a person may be diagnosed with Diabetes 2. Moderate exercise can help burn excess weight and improve the use of insulin in the body. The body requires extra fuel (glucose) during moderate exercise which will lower blood sugar. Aerobics, strength training, swimming, walking, biking in moderate amounts have all shown to be of benefit for diabetics. However, If you have been diagnosed with diabetes, please consult with your doctor on which level of exercise is appropriate, how you can monitor your insulin level, medicines and diet. According to the Center for Disease Control and Prevention's National Diabetes FACT Sheet, over 23 million people over the age of 20 were diagnosed with Diabetes 2 in 2007. This disease became the seventh leading cause of death in North America in 2006.

F. Prevent Alzheimer's

Exercise has mental benefits, too. Recent research has shown that regular exercise may not only prevent diabetes and heart disease, but it may also help prevent dementia and Alzheimer's (AD). Walking, stationary biking, gardening and swimming can help to boost the moods, keep the body strong and avoid other health problems. Since brain damage may start 10 to 20 years before an AD diagnosis, preventive measures are so important. If a family member has been diagnosed with Alzheimer's, please consult with your doctor. The National Institute of Aging states that over 4.5 million Americans have AD with that number doubling every five years because of the number of people living over the age of 65.

> *"There's clearly an inverse relationship between the amount of exercise and the number of (plaque) deposits in the brain. Exercise changes the body's reaction to forming deposits; additional blood flow to the brain may help flush away the plaque".*
>
> ~ SANGRAM SISODA ~ PROFESSOR OF NEUROSCIENCES, UNIVERSITY OF CHICAGO

Start Moving!

If you had more vitality, better health, a more positive outlook and an improved immune system, would you feel differently about yourself? If your depression lifted, heart disease, cancer, diabetes and obesity didn't exist and your energy level was higher than you could have ever imagined, how would you feel? If aches and pains disappeared and your body became stronger and more flexible, wouldn't it give you a new lease on life? It's never too late to rejuvenate ourselves; we can start now.

As mentioned above by Professor Sangram Sisoda, recent research has shown that regular exercise may not only prevent diabetes and heart disease, but actually help prevent dementia and Alzheimer's.

Those benefits alone make it all worthwhile. But before you join your local fitness center and dive into a new exercise program, check with your health practitioner, especially if you haven't been physically active in awhile.

Get Moving!

As we age, our metabolism slows. To remain fit, we need to balance daily exercise, a healthy diet (preferably full of alkaline foods), proper rest, and joyful intentions. Bob Greene, Oprah Winfrey's trainer, has this to say about what constitutes overall fitness. "Functional fitness is a person's ability to first perform exercises and movements effectively; cardio and muscle training comprises the other two-thirds of an overall fitness program."

Core training, strengthening, aerobics and flexibility are my key areas of focus. I rarely get injured or sore, I sleep better, and my weight stays where I want it. Depression lifts and life is exhilarating. Feeling sexy and desirable in the later years is an added bonus. Why not?

Getting Started

1. Be Patient

When you make a commitment to exercising, you will find the first two weeks are the biggest hurdle. Muscle soreness or just plain weariness may discourage you from sticking with your program. If you manage to exercise for just one month, you have a much better chance of staying with it for life. When you have reached the one-month benchmark, re-evaluate your regimen and see how you can perform in different and more challenging ways.

2. Start With Something You Enjoy

It could be as simple as a 15-minute walk three times a week, building up to a 30-minute walk five days a week. Don't try to start at the top; building up to 30 minutes of exercise a day is safer and encourages you to stay consistent. Years ago, Jane Fonda, along with other fitness instructors, advocated continuing the workout to the point of exhausting the muscles, thus the feeling of muscles "burning." That "burn theory" is now passé. You will not receive any more benefits working out for an hour than you will for 30 minutes.

3. Join a Club/Find a Partner

I encourage you to join a club in your neighborhood rather than investing in expensive equipment for your home that will likely wind up decorating your garage or basement. Also, working out with other people can be stimulating. The "buddy system" should encourage both of you to show up and help you keep to your regimen.

One of the most challenging parts of exercise is sticking with a program and feeling good about reaching certain goals—be it weight loss, strength and flexibility, exercising your heart and circulatory system, or simply "getting in shape."

4. Consider a Personal Trainer

A good fitness club (including your local YMCA) employs professional trainers who will help you develop a fitness regimen tailored to your needs. So, make a plan; work with a trainer three to five times when you begin. If you suffer from arthritis or other joint problems, begin your fitness program with a qualified person trained in physical therapy who has a good overall knowledge of arthritis and other joint problems.

If a personal trainer is not the way you wish to initially start, familiarize yourself with the equipment, ask questions and by all means join others in core training, yoga or Pilates classes. You will learn more about your body, have fun with others and be inspired to continue on your quest to becoming a healthier person.

5. Mix It Up

Variety is the spice of life. I see the same people doing the same exercises over and over and they look bored to tears while they talk on their cell phones. My suggestion is to try different things and decide which ones you delight in. I enjoy cross-training, which I call "mixing it up." One day I may decide to go for a swim on the day I normally take a fitness class. I don't get bored and my body says, "Oh, this is something new." It's super beneficial and so enjoyable.

6. Ways to Exercise

There are multitudes of ways to exercise. In the age of super technology, the latest invention is the Wii™ video game with workouts and balance choices. For instance, I watched a granddaughter play singles tennis with her younger sister using a control to hit the ball back and forth on the court. In my day, I needed an actual racquet, court, outfit and partner to play the game.

I purchase yoga and Pilates DVDs on the internet. They come in handy when I wish to fit in a workout without going out my front door. This section will give you a taste of different forms of exercise and their benefits. I'll cover workout equipment, Pilates, walking, yoga, water aerobics, dance and tai-chi.

What to Eat When Exercising

Exercising on an empty stomach can cause glucose stores to become low and create low blood sugar (hypoglycemia) which may result in dizziness or headaches. You risk breaking down muscle protein to provide needed carbohydrates to your body during exercise. Before your workout, bread, cereal and fruit provide the energy needed for an hour workout. If your workout is longer, within an hour following a workout, make a whey protein drink which contains 20 grams (g) whey protein. It is most important to consume whey protein immediately after your exercise session to make sure adequate protein is available to depleted muscles. Another protein suggestion is a turkey, tomato, lettuce sandwich to help rebuild muscle tissue and stimulate the immune system. Don't forget to re-hydrate with water.

A. Aerobic and Anaerobic Demystified

Aerobic exercise, such as running, provides more oxygen to your muscles and burns more calories than weight lifting. Aerobic exercise includes endurance activities such as marathon running or distance biking, walking, swimming, and cross-country skiing. Aerobic exercise also reduces chances of hip fractures, improves circulation, increases lung capacity and lowers blood pressure. It helps to increase the size of the heart muscle while providing a lower resting heart rate, thereby benefiting the entire cardiovascular system and reducing cardiovascular disease. Aerobic exercising for 20 to 30 minutes three to four times a week reduces body fat and the risk of diabetes. It also increases HDL (good) cholesterol, decreases LDL (bad) cholesterol, and promotes a longer, healthier life.

Remember to aim at the lowest part of your target zone and gradually build up to the higher part of your target zone.

Anaerobic exercise includes weight training, tennis and sprinting. Anything that requires short bursts of high intensity exertion is considered anaerobic. Weight training, an anaerobic exercise, helps make stronger bones, increases muscle strength and mass, and reduces age-related muscle atrophy. It also contributes to weight loss, though not as much as aerobic exercise. Falls occur more frequently for those over 65, so doesn't it make sense to strengthen your muscles?

> ## Workout Drinks
>
> Sports drinks are only necessary during a workout if you are exercising for ninety minutes or longer. They maximize fluid absorption and enhance performance by delivering carbohydrates and electrolytes, the most crucial of which is sodium. Sports drinks designed for use during exercise typically contain a combination of simple carbohydrates (sucrose, glucose and fructose) and complex carbohydrates, such as glucose polymers and maltodextrins. The better-formulated drinks usually contain both, with a higher percentage of complex carbohydrates rather than simple carbohydrates.

Massage

I have had massages for many years and have friends who are certified therapists. My body has experienced Hot Stones, Rolfing, Shiatsu, Swedish, Hawaiian Lomi Lomi, Reflexology, Cranial Sacral and Tai massages. When I lived near hot springs, I would soak to loosen up tight muscles and then head for my bodywork which lasted 60 to 90 minutes. I try to schedule massages twice a month, especially when I am working hard on a book project or after a strenuous hike.

Let's Talk Massage Therapy

My dear friend, Chandler McLay, became a certified massage therapist in 1996. Her other talents include guiding women's spiritual wilderness trips and working with young people and their families regarding addiction therapy. Chandler shared with me the modalities and benefits of massage therapy:

"Massage is one of the oldest remedial techniques in dealing with healing. It is also perhaps the most natural and instinctive means to relieve pain. There are accounts of massage as a healing art going back to the Chinese Amma Techniques of 3,000 B.C. Massage is mentioned in Japanese, Indian, Greek, Roman, and Arabic histories. A review of the writings of Hippocrates indicates he believed all physicians should be trained in massage. Yet, as modern Western medicine became popular, many of these historic references to simple healing arts drifted into the background. Fortunately, they are now experiencing a long-overdue recognition of their physical, emotional, and spiritual value.

It is the responsibility of each individual to become active in his/her own healing, regardless of the modality. If you choose massage as one of your healing options, I recommend you find a reputable spa or an individual therapist recommended by a reliable friend, or go to a clinic offered by a massage school. Enjoy a one hour full-body massage. Massage may be light or very deep. What does your body need? Want? Have you experienced any injuries recently or had surgery? Are you feeling depressed, sore, too heavy, or embarrassed about the shape your body is in? All these considerations will affect the quality of your relationship to your own healing. When you find a massage therapist you feel comfortable with, you will be able to simply get more deeply in touch with yourself. Professional body work often releases old traumas and dramas; that is part of its value and healing quality. Thus, I emphasize the importance of finding a therapist with whom you feel confident and comfortable."

Paybacks for Massage

- Improved circulation
- Lymph movement
- Detoxification
- Release of lactic acid after strenuous activity
- Possible improvement of blood pressure
- Pain relief
- Relaxation
- Improved flexibility
- Lubrication and exfoliation of the skin
- Emotional release
- Spiritual connection

Once you have experienced two or three general massages, you may want to be adventurous and try other varieties of body work. Read about them, ask your massage therapist about them, ask your natural health care advisor about them and find what feels good for you.

B. Weight Training ~ Making Muscle Work for You

Muscle is metabolically active; meaning it requires a lot of calories to do its thing; we burn calories by increasing our metabolism. One hour of lifting weights can burn up to 450 calories. People who want to lose weight focus on aerobic activity, although weight training can help offset our slowing metabolism and is as productive in creating a leaner body as cardiovascular activity. While cardio training may burn more calories, weight training provides stronger muscles to help ward off osteoporosis.

I completed a six-week session of weight training at my health club while writing this book. The trainer worked with me for an hour each session. Even though I had been lifting weights and using the machines, he introduced me to an entirely new way of strengthening and shaping. I now feel more confident that I can achieve maximum benefit in a 30-45 minute workout by following his guidelines. I plan to work out with this new program for a couple of months and then may go back for another session with the trainer to see what else I can achieve.

> ### Workout Guidelines
>
> - Warm up by s t r e t c h i n g your body
> - Don't consume food while exercising
> - Drink plenty of water
> - Sign up for a training session before using the equipment, and use it wisely
> - Use stretching to cool down after workout

As we grow older, it is impossible for women to develop bulk as a man does; however, weight training helps men and women tone and shape muscles, maintain flexibility, and prevent osteoporosis.

Paybacks

- Burn calories
- Strong bones

- Flexibility
- Prevent osteoporosis

C. Walk On

This is one simple exercise you can do anywhere. During the winter months, I use the treadmill and on beautiful sunshiny days I head outside for an hour walk. According to a groundbreaking study at the Erasmus M.C. University Medical Center in Rotterdam, walking at a moderate pace for 30 minutes a day, five days a week, delays cardiovascular disease and increases your life span nearly four years. Walking helps boost the metabolism, and helps prevents colorectal cancer in men. You can walk on treadmills, bike and jogging paths, around your neighborhood, or wherever you desire. Adding light hand weights and walking at a brisk pace stimulates the metabolism, makes your muscles leaner and keeps the weight off. The cardiovascular benefits for the heart and blood are superb. There are so many benefits from so little time and energy spent. And it's so simple and fun. To lose weight and keep it off, you need to get moving. You will raise your HDL (good cholesterol) and get the blood pumping through your circulatory system. You can walk with a group or by yourself. Don't forget to bring your water bottle to stay hydrated.

Paybacks

- Helps burn fat
- Cancer preventative for healthier heart, colon, and breasts
- Makes muscles leaner
- Increases blood through your circulatory system

D. Elliptical Trainers – Anaerobic

I use this machine for at least 30 minutes or cross train 10 minutes on the elliptical, stationary bike and treadmill—providing a complete 30 minute cardio workout. For those who have not used them before, elliptical trainers or "cross trainers" look like a cross between a treadmill and a step machine. As your feet move on the pedals, your legs go through an elliptical movement, reducing pounding and stress on joints in the legs, hips and back. This machine works very well to stimulate the cardiovascular system. It strengthens the quads, hamstrings and gluteus and, if using the upper body attachments, the biceps, triceps, chest, and back.

Paybacks

- Strengthens leg muscles
- Strengthens arms, back and chest
- Raises heart rate to burn fat
- Increases oxygen level

E. Stair Stepper – Aerobic

Stair steppers, or climbers, are excellent machines to burn calories and exercise the major muscle groups of the lower body. Look for sturdy, padded handrails to help balance, electronic programs to keep you interested, and easy-to-set resistance settings. A sturdy steel or aluminum frame is a must. The best stair climbers keep your feet on an even plane with the floor at all times, allowing natural foot articulation. While there is a fundamental simplicity in the stair climbing exercise itself, add-on accessories for the upper body can provide a total body workout. Plus, stepping or climbing can be a rigorous exercise in the sheer effort it takes. An all-out workout on a stair climber can consume as much energy as you are capable of producing. Besides using it regularly, try to get the maximum benefit from the machine by taking big steps and using the handrails only for light support. For a more difficult workout, let go of the rails every now and then—but take care not to lose your balance. Users who do not grip the handrails will burn upwards of 20% more calories per workout than those who lean heavily on the rails.

Paybacks

- Burns calories
- Strengthens leg muscles
- Increases healthy heart benefits
- Promotes more oxygen to lungs

F. Treadmill

Many people like the low impact of treadmills (easier on the knees), and the fact that they let you walk about as fast as you want to, or even run. While running has been a favored activity of Americans since the 1970s, walking has come into vogue in the last several years, in part because it's an exercise that older or less-fit people can do easily.

Whether you walk or run on a treadmill, it's an activity with numerous physical benefits. Many people have gotten used to using the treadmills in their health clubs and YMCAs. Of course treadmill technology is constantly changing and improving. In the past few years, a few manufacturers have come out with treadmills featuring electric inclines that adjust automatically, based on feedback from the unit's heart-rate monitor.

Paybacks

- Great for the cardiovascular system
- Improves the heart, lungs, and circulatory system
- An efficient way to lose body fat
- Since it's a weight-bearing activity, it has musculo-skeletal benefits as well

G. Recumbent Bike

If plagued by lower back pain, consider recumbent bikes. They have cushioned chair-like seats and pedals in front which offer better support for the lower back than regular bikes. The downside is you may find yourself going more slowly and easily than you would on an upright model, which means the workout won't be as difficult. You'll need to really push yourself to stay in your target heart rate zone. I vary between the recumbent bikes and the upright stationary bikes. During the beautiful weather, I bike outside.

Paybacks

- Strengthens legs
- Cardio benefits by increasing the tension
- Burns calories
- Using light hand weights increases upper body strength

H. Yoga from the Heart

Yoga, or the Sanskrit translation "union," is an ancient practice—believed to be at least five thousand years old. During my early 30s, I was raising five young children and couldn't afford the luxury of taking formal classes, let alone find a sitter to take care of the brood. I self-practiced yoga for years before stopping in favor of distance running. When I was in my 40s my back seized up and I found myself crawling to a yoga class in California. My teacher taught the Iyengar method of yoga, which is initially learned through the in-depth study of asanas (postures) and pranayama (breath control). We used props to help open various parts of the body. I found the class extremely intense but was determined to go twice a week. At times, my lower back would ache so much I told the instructor I didn't want to continue. She assured me that if I made a commitment to stay with it, I would experience relief and improvement—which I did after four to six months. To this day, in my upper 60s, the pain has not returned.

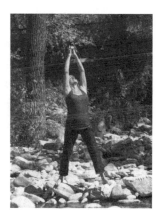

Another teacher, Hollis, recently told me that "By practicing yoga, you learn to connect with your body and listen to all of its wonderful messages. More importantly, you begin to accept the changes in your body and respect your limitations. This will be a huge lesson." My teacher's words resonate loud and clear, and I have more understanding of my injuries and the physical activities I include in my daily life. While taking a yoga class with my daughter who is in her 40s, a teacher mentioned that I was the "elder" in the room. The instructor told the vibrant men and women in their 30s that we can stay flexible our entire lives. I may be in my upper 60s, but my inner voice keeps reminding me that I still feel "youthful."

Paybacks

- Standing postures strengthen and lengthen muscles, making them less prone to injury
- Weight bearing postures help the body deposit more calcium into bones and joints
- Inverted postures direct blood and other vital fluids to specific body parts, glands, and organs and regulate hormones
- Certain postures aid in digestion and elimination

- Spine twisting postures cause the discs between the vertebrae to act as sponges soaking in blood and fluids
- Yoga's breathing techniques increases lung capacity and help quiet and focus the mind

A few words about Kundalini Yoga

I find this form of Yoga exhilarating, and practice at home for 30 to 60 minutes depending on my day. It blends well with the traditional Yoga classes. The breath work and simple movements are transformational.

Paybacks

- Teaches breathing through the nose
- Works the abdominal area
- Sends healing energy up through the spine
- Improves the function of the liver, adrenals, heart, kidneys and lungs
- Gives an inner peace and outer strength
- Creates boundless energy

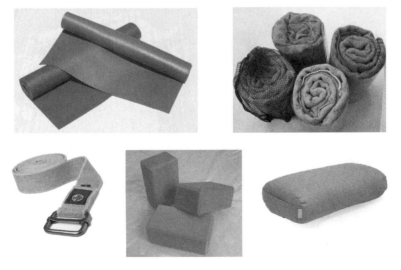

Examples of Yoga Props: Mats, Blankets, Belt, Blocks & Bolster

I. Pilates

> *"I must be right. Never an aspirin. Never injured a day in my life.*
> *The whole country, the whole world, should be doing my exercises.*
> *They'd be happier."*
>
> *- JOSEPH HUBERTUS PILATES, IN 1965, AGE 86.*

I took my first Pilates mat class when I was 59. I had heard about Pilates, but frankly didn't know what to expect. I liked it, however, and continued on with other teachers taking a variety of classes: mat, ballet routines and the reformer machine. I have been athletic my entire life, and relied on my muscles and not my core strength. Pilates was a major wake-up call for strengthening my postural muscles which include muscles that wrap around your torso. It has made me more aware of my body and how it moves. I truly love doing Pilates. I take mat classes twice a week and use resistance tools such as the magic circle and resistance bands. Recently I have started reformer classes again which consists of pulleys and springs that activate muscles differently than on the mat. When I lived in Hawaii my instructor was struck by a car while on her motorcycle, fracturing her fibula in two places and her tibia in two. Thanks to Pilates, she had an almost full recovery and was teaching one week after she left the hospital. She told me that Pilates has led her to an amazing way of movement and philosophy of being. The German Joseph Pilates, the founder of Pilates, was a sickly child which gave him the ambition to become healthy and strong. He became a skier, gymnast, boxer, and took up yoga. He taught his exercise methods to soldiers in hospitals during World War I. In 1926, Joseph Pilates came to the United States and began teaching to ballet dancers, using mats and machines.

As with all new exercises, if you have chronic pain, please consult with your health-care practitioner before you attend a Pilates class. There are many books, tapes, and videos on the subject, but none of them can take the place of an instructor. Pilates is different in each person's body; an instructor can tell you where and how you should feel each movement. A private, one-on-one lesson with an instructor is the ideal; however, this is not an option for many—cost being one factor, and finding a qualified instructor another.

Paybacks

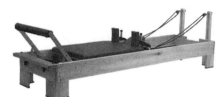

Pilates Reformer Machine

- More flexibility
- More strength
- Increased range of motion
- More abdominal strength
- Better body awareness and coordination
- Total body workout
- Better posture
- More mobility
- Helps recovery from injuries

J. Water Aerobics

We're surrounded by life-giving fluid for nine months before our births, so doesn't it make sense to connect with water during our lifetime? I have been swimming since the age of three. While living in Hawaii, I swam in the beautiful Pacific Ocean. I got to witness dolphins, turtles and reef fish swimming around me. I enjoyed the therapeutic benefits of salt water as well as hot springs. Our bodies contain 70% water, so when we are immersed in water, we relax our minds and bodies and feel better. A water aerobic instructor in Hawaii shared the following with me. "People of all ages and fitness can enjoy aqua classes. The water makes the body more buoyant, so we experience less stress on the joints. Therefore, those suffering from medical conditions such as neck or back pain, obesity, or joint aches can do the classes as well as more healthy individuals." When we are immersed in water, we reduce the pounding on bones, joints and muscles; thus we experience less soreness and pain after a class. An ideal water temperature is 83 degrees Fahrenheit.

If you are uncomfortable about using weight training equipment, aqua aerobics is an excellent alternative. Water aerobics can be done in waist-to chest-deep water, or deeper if using a flotation jacket. There are a variety of movements and programs from beginning levels to advanced. If you are new to water aerobics, let your instructor know. Schedule a time to meet with your instructor to write up a plan, whether your goal is long-term or short.

Paybacks

- Improves strength and flexibility
- Improves abdominal and back strength
- Burns an average of 450-700 calories in one hour
- Increases range of motion in knees and hips
- You can train at your own pace, eliminating the need to compete
- Safe environment for those who are not strong swimmers
- Reduces pounding of joints, bones, and muscles
- Cooler environment than on land

What to Take to the Pool

- Aqua shoes are good for traction on the pool bottom and provide more stability
- Buoys or aqua blocks (small barbells made for the water) increase resistance as you move your arms through the water
- Flotation belts help free the lower body/legs for undisturbed motion, and help with proper body alignment while in the water
- Webbed gloves increase resistance
- Kickboards are useful for lower body resistance

Safety Measures

Check with your physician before planning any exercise regime. Some health insurance companies may cover the cost of an aqua class if prescribed by a doctor. Be sure to let the instructor know if this is your first aqua class.

> *"Dancers are the Athletes of God"*
> *- ALBERT EINSTEIN*

K. Dance

I learned ballet as a child, rock and roll as a teenager, and progressed to jazz, NIA®, and Zumba® dancing as an adult.

Dance has become the rage among people of all ages, but especially Baby Boomers and older. Ballroom, hip-hop, swing, samba, tango, jazz,

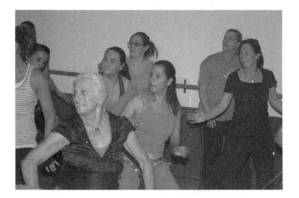

country & western, and even ballet classes are available in practically every town. Remember when dancing all night was fun and exhilarating? Dance provides so many benefits for both our physical bodies and our psyches. When we dance, we are able to lose ourselves in the rhythm and sensuous movement, leaving our troubles behind.

Zumba® is an exhilarating program. You get to boogie with easy movements to energizing music, often with Latin tempos.. In the spring of 2010, the Zumba® program had 60,000 studios in 105 countries. There are over 7.5 million participants taking Zumba classes every week.

The NIA Technique©, developed by Debbie and Carlos Rosa, provides aerobic and cardiovascular benefits, is a weight-bearing exercise, adds flexibility, and lubricates joints. Unlike many other exercise routines, dance requires no special equipment, and anyone can do it. The NIA Technique, because it is not choreographed, allows free expression in the movements. All levels are welcome.

Paybacks

- Enhances your social life
- Raises self confidence
- Helps you meet new people and make new friends
- Improves your overall heart, cardiovascular, and lung capacity
- Makes you feel more at ease in social situations
- Enhances grace and poise
- Relieves stress
- Slows aging process
- Strengthens bones, helps prevent arthritis and osteoporosis
- Burns calories
- Is just plain fun

L. Tai Chi

A few years ago, I was attending the Booksellers Association Conference in Chicago, Illinois. My hotel window overlooked Lake Michigan. One morning while preparing to go to the show, I watched a group of seniors practicing Tai Chi in a park near the lake. Their movements seemed effortless and beautiful to watch. I have taken Tai Chi lessons in nature-like settings which I find more inspirational than inside classes.

Tai Chi (tie-chee), an ancient martial art, can be performed by anyone. The slow, dance-like movement, accompanied by deep breathing, looks deceptively simple but can be a demanding, though most rewarding discipline.

One out of every three seniors will experience a fall over the course of a year. In an Emory University study, people who participated in a tai chi class once a week and practiced twice a day cut their risks of falling by 50%. Our physical strength is greatly diminished by age 50, and by age 70 we experience a one-third loss of strength in our lower extremities.

Paybacks

* Improves balance, lowers blood pressure, and reduces stress
* Helps with range of motion
* Lubricates tendons and ligaments of the lower extremities, ankles, knees, and hips
* Improves balance and coordination, bone strength, and elasticity

M. Qigong (ch'I kung)

Qigong originates from Chinese martial arts and translates as "vital energy or life force." Before becoming well known in western society, Qigong had been practiced in Buddhist and Taoist monasteries for health and spiritual benefits. In 2001 the Chinese government organized and formed the Chinese Health Qigong Association in affiliation with the Peking Sports University. Many regional colleges offer classes in Qigong as part of their school curriculum. I learned some of the movements simply because it incorporates breathing and movement techniques which flow easily and I do notice an increase in chi energy throughout my body. Persons of any age can perform these movements which contain great health and body-mind-spirit connections.

Paybacks

- Reduces stress
- Builds stamina and increases vitality
- Enhances the immune system
- Improves cardiovascular, respiratory, circulatory, lymphatic, and digestive functions

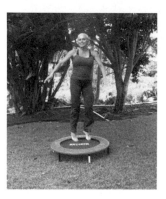

N. Rebounder/trampoline

A trampoline/rebounder provides excellent exercise and is just great fun. It stimulates all of your 75 trillion cells while strengthening your body at the same time. I have a small sturdy rebounder purchased at K-Mart for $15. I jump on it just 10 minutes a day, usually while listening to music. If you have difficulty with balance, there are rebounders with a bar you can hold onto. If you don't have a place for a small trampoline, bouncing for ten minutes while sitting on the side of your bed is also beneficial.

Paybacks

- Circulates oxygen to your tissues
- Stimulates metabolism
- Firms muscles, reducing obesity
- Provides more energy & lessens fatigue
- Improves vision
- Aids in lymphatic circulation
- Lowers cholesterol and triglycerides
- Improves digestion and elimination
- Strengthens heart and body muscles
- Increases balance and coordination
- Increases red blood cell count
- Reduces headaches and other pain
- Improves immune system
- Slows aging process

O. Inversion Table

As we age, gravity weighs us down, resulting in poor posture, weak stomach muscles (our core), and back pain. Our spine compresses, so we also become shorter by as much as two inches. It is not uncommon to see older people hunched over as if preparing to go back into the womb. Years ago, while visiting the Cayman Islands, our group took a boat trip to an outer island to visit an artist's studio. Although I was only in my early 30s at the time, one of the sculptures left an indelible impression: it was a man aging through the cycles of life, starting out as a fresh newborn, then an adult standing straight and tall, and finally ending as a crouched-over old man.

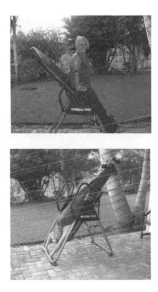

More Paybacks

- Studies have shown that within ten seconds, back pain decreases by 35%; the spine assumes its proper "S" curve and posture improves
- Helps stimulate circulation
- Helps balance awareness and motion sickness by stimulating the inner ear
- Maintains internal organs in normal position, avoiding "prolapse" (to fall out of place)
- Increases oxygen to the brain
- Helps reverse the effects of gravity
- Relieves back pain
- Reduces stress
- Strengthens and elongates the spine
- Allows more space between the vertebrae and relieves pressure on discs
- Helps relax tense muscles
- Speeds the flow of lymphatic fluids which flush out the body's wastes

and carry them to the bloodstream

• Introduces fresh supplies of oxygen

• Helps stiffness and muscle pain disappear

There are smaller inversion chairs available, and you may be able to obtain one with a physician's script and your health insurance. Always consult with a physician before you use an inversion table, especially if you have high blood pressure or other conditions.

Healthy Numbers

Dr. Mehmet Oz, Director of Cardiovascular and Complementary Medicine Program at New York-Presbyterian Hospital and author of over 400 publications and medical books, believes that these eight numbers are important to monitor for better health.

1. Blood Pressure: aim for 115/75

The average middle-age blood pressure is 130/80, which Dr. Oz says isn't good enough being that cardiovascular disease is already a major health problem.

2. Resting Heart Rate: 83

Before rising, take your pulse by placing two fingers on your carotid artery or wrist. Count beats per minute. If your resting heart rate is higher than 83, Dr. Oz says you are at a higher risk for a heart attack. In order to improve your resting heart rate it is vital to increase your physical activity. While exercising, subtract your age from 220 and multiple that number by 0.8. The final number will give you your ideal rate.

3. Cholesterol: 2 to 1

If you have a family history of high blood pressure, diabetes or if you smoke, your LDL (bad) level should be under 100. If you have none of these risk factors, between 100-129 is optimal. Your HDL (good) level should be above 60. Doctors say the measurement of LDL to HDL should be less than two to 1, though a ratio of three to 1 is still manageable.

4. Omega-6 to Omega-3s: 4 to 1

Eat more fish, whole grains, ground flaxseeds, beans and nuts. Limit processed foods and oils from safflower, corn, cottonseed and peanuts. A balance of Omega 6 and 3 will help to decrease risk of cardiovascular disease, certain cancer, arthritis and asthma.

5. Inflammation: 1

A blood test can gauge your C- reactive protein (CRP). If your number is under one, your chances of having heart disease is less than half. If the number is above 10, other ailments may be present which include autoimmune disease. For prevention, floss daily and consume more of the Mediterranean diet to include vegetables, whole grains, olive oil, fruits and an occasional glass of wine. I cannot help wondering that if this testing had been available during my mother's life, her rheumatoid arthritis may have been managed better and given her a longer life.

6. Vitamin D: 30

A blood test result should show a hydroxy level between 30 – 50. During the winter months we are exposed to less sunshine. Deficiencies may lead to multiple sclerosis, cancer, heart disease and osteoporosis. My mother also suffered from osteoporosis. Perhaps if my mother had heeded my father's wisdom to relocate to the sunny Arizona desert, she would have felt better. Lack of sunshine and the damp, cold northeastern climate made my mom's physical condition worse. Take a supplement with at least 1,000 mg of Vitamin D3 daily or cod liver oil. My grown children remember drinking cod liver oil while they were growing up. They still make faces telling me that story.

7. Blood Sugar: 125

Your blood sugar should register under 100 after an 8-hour or overnight fast. If you're not fasting, the number should be less than 125. Eat chia seeds in yogurt or salads; they help slow the rate at which sugar is absorbed.

8. Bone Density: 1

The Standard DEXA 9 dual energy X-ray absorptiometry scan gives your bone density and compares it to that of a young woman. Above one is normal; 1 to 2.5 indicates osteopenia which could lead to osteoporosis; above 2.5 indicates osteoporosis. This testing is recommended for women who are no longer on hormone replacement therapy. It is generally good to be tested around age 50 for women who have had a family history of osteoporosis or a hip fracture. To help maintain bone strength and density, take a daily dose of 1,000 IU of Vitamin D, 1200 milligrams of calcium, and 400 milligrams of magnesium and do strength and resistance training two to three days a week.

Healthier Living Beyond the Challenges

Stanford University's Patient Education Research Center has developed a project called "Healthier Living with Ongoing Health Problems." This program currently is implemented in 16 states and 17 countries. 1,000 participants were involved in a five-year research project that showed that people who attended the program improved their health behaviors through exercise, cognitive symptom management, coping, and better communication with physicians. They also noticed a decrease in fatigue and distress as well as a significant decline in the duration of hospital stays.

If you are concerned about diabetes, arthritis, heart disease or other chronic health conditions, you might want to consider taking this course. It is also offered online.

The Blue Zones

For five years, Dan Buettner, along with National Geographic, National Institute of Aging, European demographers, medical scientists and journalists, researched four regions of the world where people live longer and healthier lives. The survey included lifestyle, diet, medicines, socialization and physical activity. These places were coined the blue zones. There is a three times better chance of these blue zone cultures becoming centenarians (100 years of age or older).

Loma Linda, California USA

This town contains a large community of Seven Day Adventists. They are a devout group who have a large and supportive community which supports one another culturally and socially.

Seven Day Adventists

Their foods are plant based from grains and seeds and inspired from the Book of Genesis. Saturdays are their Sabbath or which they call the "sanctuary in time." Their life expectancy is 9 to 11 years longer than their American counterparts.

Sardinia, Italy

This is the next stop in the fountain of youth tour. Sardinia is an island off the coast of Italy. There are more male centenarians living here than anywhere else in the world.

Italians

Giovanni Sannai, 104 years old, chops wood and has his morning glass of red wine rich in antioxidants. He proceeded to beat Buettner in a round of arm wrestling.

This sounds like a good life to me. Also, on Sardinia, the elders are greatly respected, a contrast to our culture in America where many elders are forgotten.

Nicoya Peninsula, Costa Rica

The Nicoya Peninsula on the west coast of Costa Rica is a third blue zone where people live to a ripe old age surpassing 100. A traditional day for Panchita, who is deaf and partially blind and celebrated her 100th birthday in 2008, would be rising at 4:00 a.m. praying, and gathering up her chicken eggs, grinding corn by hand, making coffee, and gathering her water from the nearby well. Her breakfast meal consists of tortillas, eggs, and beans. They grow their own gardens for fresh

Costa Ricans

They live simply without adding stress to their daily lives. Passed down by indigenous roots of the Chorotega, they exhibit a low rate of heart disease, and have strong bones and hips, which may be attributed to their drinking water source containing high amounts of calcium.

food. She then splits wood and clears bush away from her modest home. Her son is 80; a great-grandfather who still exudes plenty of energy. The Nicoyan community is a close-knit group where families live together, have a strong support system among their friends, and display the belief that they will always be taken care of by God no matter what challenges may arise in their lives.

Japanese

Their diet consists of several servings of fruits and vegetables each day. Fish is consumed several times a week. They are physically active and involved in numerous activities such as walking, gardening, dancing, and karate all performed without going to a gym.

Okinawa, Japan

The last stop along the road to longevity is Okinawa, the main island off the coast of Japan. This area holds the current world record for life span with the average age of women at 85 and men 78 years of age. There are over 457 centenarians on Okinawa and most people who live the longest are free of disabilities. Also the 80 and 90 year olds are as healthy and active as people 30 years younger.

The people of Okinawa have a strong sense of community and family, have healthy habits and are relatively free of stress unlike most of the world. Their life purpose, faith, and perhaps their affinity toward mugwort sake may give them healthier years ahead.

Genes may play a 50% part in our destiny. However, if we mirror different lifestyle choices that are similarly reflected in the blue zones, such as: aging gratefully, gracefully and healthfully, we can gift ourselves a longer and happier life. This chapter has presented you with oodles of exercise suggestions. It does take discipline and an awareness of our body and our health. Even my grandmother, with only one leg, managed to walk each day. Take the steps to physically be the best person you can be, and you will reap huge rewards.

> *"If we could give every individual the right amount of nourishment and exercise, not too little and not too much, we would have found the safest way to health"*
>
> ~ *HIPPOCRATES*

— Step 3 —

Nutrition:
We Are What We Eat

When I prepared meals for my five children, we had at least one meal a day in which we would eat slowly and consciously and say a prayer to give thanks for the food before us, the love between us and the friends around us. Those meals became our sharing time. We didn't rush. Sitting around our dining room table we were together as a family; sharing our day, laughing and coming together to appreciate one another. As a child, I had Sunday dinners with our grandparents in a similar manner. The meals stretched out for hours while we practically worshipped the Italian cuisine lavishly prepared by my grandmother, aunt and mother. The food was always prepared fresh and in great abundance with ingredients bought from the local Italian grocery stores. On holidays and special occasions we had Italian ham (prosciutto) laced over melon slices, antipasto, escarole soup, pasta with homemade marinara sauce and meatballs made from beef, pork and veal, fresh meats or fowl, cheeses, salads, Italian breads; and always the irresistible Italian deserts served with coffee and anisette and hard cookies to dip into the coffee. The Chianti bottle was passed around the table, and there were bottles of soda for the children. Afterwards, the men would rest in the living room while the women cleaned the dishes and the children ran outside to play.

In 1989, the Slow Food movement began to counteract fast food and fast life. It is now in 32 countries. This non-profit organization introduces origins of local food and the joy of eating foods from various regions around the world. We were living the slow food movement years before it became the thing to do.

Foods and Your Health

Did you know that the top three diseases in the U.S—heart disease, cancer and diabetes—can be directly linked to diet? Almost two-thirds of the population of the United States, and over one billion of the world's population, is now considered overweight. This is at an all-time high. 300 million people worldwide are classified as obese. We know that obesity is a causative factor in many diseases, diabetes among them. One in three children born today will have diabetes in their lifetime.

Alzheimer's disease, which affects over 4.5 Americans and 24 million worldwide, is also impacted by diet. According to a recent study published in the Annals of Neurology (2006, vol. 59, no. 6), an emphasis on a Mediterranean diet consisting of fruits, vegetables, whole grains, olive oil and fish reduced the risks of Alzheimer's. According to a Columbia University study, people who adhered to the Mediterranean diet had a 40% lower risk of Alzheimer's than those who did not adhere to the diet.

What we eat is vitally important to both preventing and reversing disease and maintaining our good health. The current health-care system in America does not promote disease prevention, simply because health care providers are in the business of treating sickness. The pharmaceutical industry, food producers, and restaurants are all in business to make money. It is up to us to decide what is good for us and take responsibility for our overall health. Don't stress about food. Remember, nutrition plays a vital role in our lives. If you overeat, under-eat, or feel guilty about what you eat, you won't be doing yourself any favors. So relax about your intake and know that you will make wiser food choices as your body becomes stronger and leaner.

Paybacks

Boost Metabolism

As we continue to age, our metabolism slows down as much as 20 to 40%. Metabolic Syndrome makes a person more susceptible to diabetes, heart disease and strokes. Over 47 million Americans have been diagnosed with Metabolic Syndrome; people who are overweight and obese are more likely to develop the syndrome.

Healthy foods and regular exercise can assist in boosting a sluggish metabolism. Add a variety of fresh fruits, nuts, eggs, vegetables and fiber to your daily diet. Enrich your diet by including Omega-3 foods, salmon and tuna. Omega-3 rich foods can boost our metabolism to help burn calories. Avoid processed foods and fast food restaurants.

A Healthier Heart

Many people have unhealthy diets filled with saturated fats including white flour, donuts, cakes, pies, cold cuts, bacon, breaded and fried meats, full fat dairy products, canned fruits and fried vegetables as examples. The result is a high probability of coronary artery heart disease, high blood cholesterol, and high triglycerides.

Introduce healthier foods. Monounsaturated fats and polyunsaturated fats can assist in lowering blood cholesterol. Eat low-fat proteins which include low-fat dairy products, egg whites, skinless chicken, and free-range meat. Include fresh fruits and vegetables and whole grains, reduce salt consumption and make food portions smaller.

Lower Cholesterol

Cholesterol is a type of fat. In the previous chapter, we have discussed the two types: the "good fat," high density lipoprotein (HDL) and the "bad fat," low density lipoprotein (LDL). Triglyceride is also another lipid (fat) which should be monitored. Remember the Duke University Medical Center and East Carolina University study? Overweight people who exercised at least 30 minutes a day were able to lower their LDL. The ones who added more vigorous exercise such as up to 20 miles a week of jogging not only lowered LDL but also increased HDL rates.

Begin by including unsaturated fats: soybean, sesame and olive oils to name a few. Be wary of commercial dressings which may also contain saturated fats. Egg yolks, some shellfish, high-fat dairy products, organ meats and poultry all contain cholesterol. Vegetables, nuts, seeds, fruits and grains do not contain cholesterol. Oats, barley, oranges, apples and beans may help to decrease cholesterol amounts. Plain complex carbohydrate foods like rice, pasta and potatoes can be included without adding creams or rich sauces.

Prevent Joint Pain/Arthritis

People who weigh 20% or more than their "normal" weight are more likely to place more stress on knees, hips, legs, spine, and feet. My mother was treated for her rheumatoid arthritis with corticosteroid therapy. There were days her feet were so swollen she couldn't walk. After several years of receiving multiple cortisone shots and gold injections, her hands and feet still became permanent twisted shapes. Arthritis drug side effects may increase appetite, promote weight gain and produce fluid retention. Osteoarthritis may also contribute to weight gain.

Throughout the years, people with arthritis have complained of joint swelling and pain after consuming eggplant, potatoes, tomatoes and peppers, all from the nightshade family. Sugar, red meat, chocolate, salt, additives and preservatives may also be contributing factors. There is little research connected to diet and arthritis. However, eating cold water fish like salmon, sardines and trout which contain high levels of Omega-3's may aid in reducing inflammation within the body. Drinking three to four cups of green tea (polyphenolic compounds) a day may also help to decrease certain RA symptoms.

Prevent Alzheimer's

Alzheimer's research has been discussed in the "mind" section of this book.

Nutrition plays an important role in keeping our brains smart and Alzheimer's at bay. Have a healthy, well balanced diet, limit sugar and salt intake and drink eight glasses of water a day. Eggs are rich in acetylcholine, a neurotransmitter. Low levels of this have been linked to patients with Alzheimer's. Salads are packed with antioxidants to help ward off free radicals from forming and help provide better cognitive skills. Yogurt contains tyrosine, an amino acid, which helps our memory and alertness. There are complications that arise if a person is in a more aggressive stage of Alzheimer's. When the nerve cells die off, a person may lose interest in food, have difficulty eating and not recognize whether or not they are hungry or thirsty. At this stage, medical supervision is vitally important.

Inflammation

Dr. West, referring to in the supplement section, says that inflammation occurs through cell damage and eating wrong foods: sugar, processed, charbroiled and barbequed foods, pasta, breads, pastries and baked goods which can increase levels of pro-inflammatory peptides. Our organs directly benefit from a healthy inflammatory process.

Suggestions include vegetables, olive and coconut oil, flax seeds and nuts, and aloe vera juice. Eat fish high in Omega-3's twice a week and ingest or cook with olive, hempseed, flax, grapeseed, rice bran, coconut or walnut oils. Green, orange and yellow vegetables, blueberries, spinach, soy milk, and tofu all have anti-inflammatory properties.

Diabetes

Over 23 million people in America have been diagnosed with diabetes. Worldwide the statistics are at 246 million people. That number will rise by the year 2025 to 385 million people, making the disease a worldwide epidemic. Type 1 Diabetes occurs among younger people, and is commonly treated with insulin injections. Type 2 ,which affects 90% of those diagnosed with diabetes, occurs after age 40 and can often be treated through exercise, diet, and medication.

If you have been diagnosed with diabetes, ask yourself, "What foods help to control my blood sugar, blood pressure and help keep cholesterol levels in a healthy range?"

Maintaining a diet which contains 70% alkalized foods helps keep the PH levels healthy. Dark green leafy vegetables and salads assist in helping rid the body of acid-forming chemicals. Limit unhealthy fats, sugary sweets, and add more fiber and low glycemic foods which consist of protein, low glycemic carbohydrates and Omega-3 foods. A low glycemic plan helps to keep energy high during exercise, maintains healthy weight and cholesterol levels and increases insulin resistance. There are charts on the Internet which list low glycemic foods.

My Kitchen Secrets

At one time or another I have joined an organic co-op to stock my kitchen with raw yogurt, milk, cream, cheese, and local vegetables and fruits. I was a vegetarian for many years; however, because I am physically active and live at a higher altitude, I made the change to eat high-quality protein. I eat very little red meat, but when I do it's organic, and usually buffalo or elk. I only eat organic fowl. Cold water fish such as halibut or salmon are eaten twice a week. Usually I have smaller portions of protein mixed with larger portions of vegetables. Basically, I purchase locally grown pesticide-free or organic fruits, vegetables, grains, nuts, and fish.

I focus on keeping my diet 80% alkaline and 20% acid. If the body becomes too acidic, health issues can arise. I encourage you to purchase Shelley Young's recipe books. The meals are simple and good and will help familiarize you with eating alkalized foods.

Breakfast

I will eat a small serving of buckwheat, oatmeal or quinoa, adding a small amount of raw almond butter which is ground in my Vitamix, slivers of apple, banana, strawberries or blueberries and ground flax seed. I include walnuts which are high in essential fatty acids, or raw almonds which I soak in water and place in a jar in my refrigerator, making them more digestible. Consume the nuts within two days. Eating complex carbohydrates an hour before a workout or class is very beneficial. It provides energy. For sweeteners, I use a packet of Stevia which is a natural sweetener and safe for diabetics. The more alkaline the body becomes, the more the craving for donuts, breads, sweets and processed foods disappears. If I am headed to an exercise class, I take a bottle of water and add a teaspoon of powdered greens and vitamin C. This drink is packed with protein, enzymes, amino acids and keeps me hydrated.

Late Morning Post-Workout

I prepare a protein meal which helps rebuild muscle I have spent during my workout routine. I am not a fan of protein bars; although I understand their concept if you are participating in a run or bike race or other high-energy activities. I concentrate on feeding my body with organic healthy sources which include farm fresh eggs, organic unsweetened yogurt or a protein drink with lecithin, banana, blueberries and flax oil.

Lunch

This is a great time for me to get my live (not cooked) foods. I make a large salad of organic greens, dark leafy vegetables, carrots, tomatoes, avocado, celery, cucumbers, sprouts, pumpkin seeds, and tofu; or if you are not yet a tofu lover, add a small amount of coldwater fish such as trout, salmon, sardines or cod. This is my high-protein meal in the middle of the day when my metabolism is high and my system can easily digest the food. My energy level stays high and I am satisfied until mid afternoon.

Mid-afternoon Snack

Raw nuts such as almonds, hazelnuts, pecans, pistachios, pumpkin and sunflower are especially nutritious and alkaline. It's a good idea to soak these nuts, which helps to activate the enzymes, making them easier to digest and increases the nutritional value. Cover nuts with water and refrigerate the container for an hour (overnight for almonds). Rinse and eat within two days to prevent mold from forming.

Another treat could be an Ezekiel™ tortilla located in many health food and grocery stores in the refrigerator section. Mash up an avocado with tomatoes and spread on the tortilla.

Dinner

This meal should be eaten at least three hours before bedtime. Our metabolism slows down as we approach the end of the day, so in order to digest food properly, do not eat too late in the evening. The adage "Eat like a king in the morning, a queen in the afternoon, and a prince in the evening" does contain powerful wisdom.

I enjoy warming foods at this time; vegetable soups, lightly steamed vegetables, rice or quinoa. Before bed, I prepare herbal tea or warmed soymilk or almond milk sprinkled with cinnamon, and I sleep like a princess without the pea.

Eating Tips

> *"When diet is wrong, medicine is of no use. When diet is correct, medicine is of no need."*
>
> ~ *AYURVEDIC SAYING*

If your kitchen has been stocked with fresh whole foods, you are well on your way to vibrant health. Your body and mind will be happier for feeding it well. Food which is locally grown and free of pesticides and sprays should always be your number one choice. I like to prepare my produce when I bring it home by washing it, cutting it and placing it in refrigerated containers. I do not refrigerate my tomatoes; and some of the bananas get peeled and go into a freezer bag. I use them for my protein drinks. Here are several tips for healthy eating;

- Eat whole foods that have not been chemically sprayed, and always rinse your produce with a fruit/vegetable product which removes any remaining chemicals and sprays
- Avoid corn syrup, food colorings, monosodium glutamate and other artificial additives
- Season with garlic, turmeric, kelp, seaweed, cinnamon, cayenne pepper, and sesame seeds
- Avoid sugar, too much caffeine, and any processed foods
- Avoid getting your carbohydrates from refined foods high in sugar; eat only complex carbohydrates
- Indulge in raw and lightly steamed vegetables, tofu, small quantities of cold-water fish (twice weekly), garlic, fresh grains, legumes, nuts and seeds, sprouts, tomatoes, avocados, lemons, limes and grapefruit, and at least 60 ounces of purified water a day. Greens contain more than enough to meet the body's protein requirements (elephants and gorillas eat only grass and leaves and look at their strength); eating hot peppers can relieve cluster, migraine and sinus headaches
- Buy free range organic meat or fowl only; you will be consuming a product which the animal did not receive hormones, arsenic or antibiotics
- Consume foods that contain antioxidants, including leafy greens, broccoli, spinach, kale, nuts, apples, blueberries, cherries, grapes and even Spirulina; all of which support the body, ward off senility, and fuel the brain. Our brains contain high levels of fat; when we eat the wrong kinds of food, free radicals attach to the fat
- Eat small meals during the day, eat only when hungry, and slowly chew your food. This can help keep our metabolism charged and keep the pounds off. The Center for Disease Control recommends 1600 calories a day for women and 1900 for men. According to The Journal of the American Medical Association (JAMA), cutting down on daily food intake can extend your life
- Eat locally-grown foods that are in season. When I was living in Hawaii, seasons were very subtle, but I still found myself eating warming soups and more grains and proteins during the winter months when the temperatures were lower. In the spring, add greens,

berries and sprouts, and in the summer months eat more fresh vegetables, greens, carbohydrates and fruits which help to detoxify the body and supply needed energy

- Have your main meal in the middle of the day; your muscles are strong in the morning, but in the middle of the day your digestion is strongest
- Eat breakfast, lunch and dinner, and eat sensibly for your weight and size
- Eat slowly in a quiet, tension-free environment
- Avoid snacking or grazing during the day, especially on sugar and simple carbohydrates such as chips
- Avoid trendy diets that may initially appear to be working but eventually become more detrimental to your physical balance, producing fatigue, stress, depression and high acidity which will cause your weight to yo-yo
- Slow down; when we eat on the run, we usually down empty calories and deny our bodies wholesome nutritional antioxidant-packed foods

Should My Food Be Cooked or Raw?

I feel better when I eat 70 to 80% raw or lightly steamed foods. I also like to lightly steam vegetables to go along with my salad. Too much cooked food slows my digestion and makes me feel sluggish. Dr. Gabriel Cousens recommends taking a B12 supplement if you don't eat animal protein.

Benefits of Eating Live Food

- Lower cholesterol and tri-glycerides
- Lower incidences of stomach cancer
- Build a stronger immune system

Some foods retain more of their nutrients when cooked,

Results of Cooking Food

When we heat food over 114 degrees, it destroys live enzymes and destroys up to 80% of vitamins and minerals. According to Gabriel Cousens, M.D., "You lose more than ninety percent of a food's B12, half of the protein, and one hundred percent of enzymes and phytonutrients."

such as cabbage and tomatoes, although grains and beans are more acidic when cooked. If your diet consists mainly of cooked foods, you can slowly introduce raw or live food to your meals. For instance, at lunch time, have a salad along with your protein source. Eventually you will begin to eliminate cooked foods and find yourself eating carrot or celery sticks dipped in guacamole. Your system will become more alkaline and your cravings for gooey processed foods and sweets will be greatly diminished. You will be sending different "messages" to your body and over time it will become part of your lifestyle.

Safe Cookware

- Ceramic enameled cookware has good heat distribution, is dishwasher friendly, and easy to clean and maintain
- Copper cookware is lined with tin or stainless steel to keep copper from getting into foods; the pots have even heat distribution, but keeping my copper pots shined up was a task
- Stainless steel cookware is made up of small amounts of different metals and safe to cook with
- Aluminum cookware is now anodized which makes it safe and non - stick and scratch resistant; this is my current choice
- Teflon cookware is relatively safe and the Environmental Protection Agency (EPA) says the small Teflon flaking doesn't affect our health; if you are unsure about Teflon, do some research
- Cast iron pots and pans are excellent to have in your kitchen; they need to be seasoned and washed without soap; I used mine for years at home and for camping

Water

How much pure water do you consume each day? How pure is your water source? If you are not a "water person," or if you wait to drink water when you are thirsty, chances are you are already in a state of dehydration. If you exercise and sweat or live in a humid climate which causes you to perspire, and you do not drink adequate amounts of water, chances are you are very dehydrated.

A good rule of thumb is to drink at least 64 ounces of good water daily.

Better yet, drink 10 to 12 eight-ounce glasses daily. As we've mentioned, soft drinks and caffeinated beverages will dehydrate our bodies. Many of us fill up on soda, juice, teas and alcoholic beverages, so we don't have room for pure water. Maybe we don't like the taste of water by itself and want to add something to it to make it more palatable. It's important that we break ourselves of this habit and learn to love the taste of pure water.

On the flip side, too much water can be dangerous as well. Athletes who constantly drink large amounts of water can experience a condition called hyponatremia, where salt levels in the blood fall dangerously low. That's why it's important to consume electrolytes if you are exercising, running, or working out and consuming large quantities of water.

What is Safe Drinking Water?

During the 1990's my publishing company, Kali Press, came out with a book titled *"Don't Drink the Water (without reading this book): The Essential Guide to Our Contaminated Drinking Water and What You Can Do about It"* by Lono A'o. The book lists the health hazards involved in drinking public as well as ground water. It highlights the many contaminants that are put into our public water systems and the chemicals being dumped into the soil which then leach into the groundwater. We also see more contaminants such as gas leaks, pesticides and pharmaceutical drugs leaching into the soil and eventually into the groundwater. Such is the case in California where high levels of TCE contamination have become a major health hazard in certain areas. California is not alone in this epidemic. Stronger standards need to be enforced on local, state and federal levels. Besides a link to cancer and the nervous system, contaminants also can disrupt our hormonal balance. This is not a pretty picture.

Although I am not a trained scientist, my research throughout the years has led me to understand that certain public water systems, untested wells, living around chemical plants or large industrial complexes and certain bodies of water all may be a contributing factor in our poor health. Meanwhile what can you do to obtain better drinking water? The bottled water industry has exploded. It seems every time you go to the supermarket there is another brand of bottled drinking water on the shelf. Now we can choose between spring water, distilled water, natural artesian water, mountain spring water, alpine spring water, and many more to add to the confusion. Bottled water doesn't have to comply with stringent testing guidelines, so what you think you are drinking may not necessarily be the best water.

It's also a good idea to drink water from glass or stainless containers. Drinking water from a plastic bottle which has been exposed to high heat (perhaps while in your car) is not advisable as certain toxins from the plastics can leach into the water. Various plastics leach a chemical called bisphenol (BPA) which mimic female hormone estrogen. In the U.S.A over 90% of Americans age six and up have experienced higher levels of BPA which may lead to obesity, infertility and some forms of cancer. Avoid plastic bottles which have the number three, six and seven on the bottom and consider purchasing stainless bottles. Kleankanteen.com sells 100% recycled food grade stainless drinking containers for adults and children.

Choosing a Water Filter

In order to filter out harmful substances in your water you can test your water for chlorine, lead, mercury, aluminum, cadmium, chromium, copper, bacteria, viruses and radioactive material such as Radon and Uranium. There are filtration systems which range in choices from pitchers to counter top, under sink purifiers and full house systems. Don't forget to research shower and tub filters while you are at it The skin is our largest organ, after all, and absorbs everything. I have a water filter at my kitchen sink and a shower filter to eliminate public water additives. I have a large crock pot with a spigot in which I store my drinking water.

First-Rate Fats

We have become a low- and no-fat society, but this is not particularly healthy. Eating fats that do not clog the arteries is the key to getting proper nutritional values from fats. About 20% of your diet should be made up of healthy fats. What are some of those good fats?

- Polyunsaturated fats such as evening primrose, flaxseed, grape seed, and borage are all available in capsules or gel caps. These fats help the body eliminate acids, regulate hormones, and develop healthy cells
- Monounsaturated fats include olive oil, raw nuts and avocados; these fats increase your energy and contribute to healthy, vibrant skin
- Essential fatty acids—these are the good fats which the body achieves through your diet; they are long-chain poly-unsaturated acids which include Omega-3, 6 and 9. Essential fatty acids are necessary to ele-

vate mood, provide beautiful skin, increase a healthy immune system, support mental clarity and normalize weight (you need to eat fat to burn fat). They produce prostaglandins which support healthy heart function, blood pressure and blood clotting

Brands - Uses and Storage

Some brands recommended for supplemental oils are: Udo's Choice,* Barlean's Organic Oils,* and Omega Nutrition,* all available in health food stores and food markets.

Do not heat these oils. Add them to salads, smoothies or to cooked vegetables. Store your oils in a place away from heat after opening.

Benefits of Flax:

Lignans provide up to 700 times the amount of fiber found in legumes or whole grains which help prevent certain cancers.

One tablespoon of flaxseed oil will provide the daily amount of linolenic acid. Whole flaxseed can be put in a grinder. Store it in a sealed glass container in your refrigerator. Use it in smoothies, protein drinks, on cereal and in plain yogurt. Flaxseed can be sprinkled on any food.

- Rich in Omega-3's and lignans which are natural antioxidants
- Helps prevent heart disease
- Helps remove toxins
- Helps allergies and digestive problems
- Provides healthy skin, hair and nails
- Better brain development
- More rapid healing
- Improves athletic performance

Coconut Oil

Coconut oil contains high levels of lauric acid, which makes it an excellent preventative for heart disease. Its antiviral, anti-fungal, antimicrobial and anti-tumor properties lower blood cholesterol and arterial plaque as well as strengthen the immune system. Coconut oil also stimulates metabolism and activates normal thyroid function, which does decline with age. It contains medium-chain fatty acids, which are more easily digested and metabolized in the body. I cook with coconut oil. It has a high smoke point of 350 degrees replacing many oils including olive oil. Olive oil is great uncooked as in a salad dressing, or drizzled over vegetables. I purchase high quality organic coconut oil. It keeps forever without refrigeration. It is a great substitute for people who have nut allergies. Your body will love three and a half tablespoons of coconut oil per day (melt and consume), or you can drink 10 ounces of coconut milk to get the same benefit.

Coconut Oil Suggestions

- Popcorn: add two tablespoons of coconut oil and a quarter cup popcorn kernels to a pan over medium to high heat; cover, shake the pan to evenly distribute the kernels
- Oatmeal: stir one tablespoon into hot oatmeal and sprinkle with cinnamon
- Smoothie: add one tablespoon into soy or almond milk; add one frozen banana, blueberries, and blend

Recipes

Veggie - Flax Burgers

1 6.5 ounce jar artichoke hearts, drained and quartered
1 teaspoon chopped garlic
¼ cup chopped green onions
3 tablespoons chopped fresh parsley, or 2 teaspoons dried
¾ cup cooked garbanzo beans, drained and rinsed
¾ cup cooked kidney bean or black beans, drained and rinsed
3 tablespoons ground flaxseed, regular or golden
2 tablespoons roasted tahini or other nut butter
4 generous twists of black pepper
½ cup cooked brown rice or millet
Cooking spray
4 whole grain hamburger buns (optional)

1. Place artichoke hearts, garlic, green onions, parsley, garbanzo beans, kidney or black beans, ground flaxseed, sesame tahini, and pepper in a

food processor; pulse about 8 times, until blended. Scrape down sides and pulse another 6 times. Do not over process. Transfer to a bowl and gently stir in cooked rice or millet.

2. Divide mixture into 4 portions and form into patties ½ inch thick.

3. Heat a large nonstick frying pan over medium heat and coat with cooking spray. Fry burgers until bottoms are brown, about 5 minutes. Spray tops of burgers with cooking spray and flip. Cook until brown, about 5 minutes. Serve on buns if desired.

4. Per serving: 215 cal, 37% fat cal, 9g fat, 1g sat fat,10g protein, 24g carb, 9g fiber, 331 mg sodium.

I have made these burgers many times and found them yummy and a terrific substitute for a meat burger. You can use lean meat like buffalo or elk if you have meat eaters in your family. This recipe has protein, fiber and the benefits of healthy fats. Try it with lettuce, sliced tomato, and avocado.

Avocados

Avocados contain 10 to 15% protein and little sugar (about 2%). They are loaded with minerals, including iron, copper and more potassium than bananas (which are high in sugar). They contain a high quality fat which quickly satisfies hunger. Eating avocados improves your red blood cells, and the lutein in avocados helps to protect against cancer and eye diseases.

I eat at least one avocado a day, although two or three are very beneficial and will not make you put on extra weight. Do not combine them with proteins or melons.

Avocado - Sprout Salad

2 cups sprouts
½ cup diced celery
½ cup diced red onion
½ cup thinly sliced carrots
1 red pepper, diced
4 teaspoons lemon juice
2 teaspoons dulse flakes

1-2 avocados

In a small bowl, combine the sprouts, celery, onion, carrots, red pepper, lemon juice and dulse. Toss thoroughly. Add the avocados and mix gently. Serve on a lettuce leaf. Serves 2. *Recipe from "The Raw Gourmet" by Nomi Shannon.*

Goat Cheese

For people who are lactose intolerant, goat cheese is a great substitute for regular cheese, making it more tolerable and digestible. It is also lower in fat and calorie content. It provides a great source of calcium, boosts metabolism, is easy to digest, and is high in protein. It contains potassium, vitamin A, selenium, niacin and tryptophan. One of my granddaughters is lactose intolerant; however, she can digest goat's milk and cheese. I enjoy it sprinkled in salads and in an appetizer spread in lieu of cream cheese. Try it on pizzas and in pasta dishes.

Other Healthy Foods to Consider

Quinoa

Quinoa, once a staple food of the Inca civilization, is now considered the super grain. It is a complete protein and provides all eight essential amino acids as well as minerals, B vitamins and fiber. Quinoa can be purchased at any health food store, specialty food store and some grocery chains. I enjoy eating it warm, but it also makes a delightful cold salad. Here is one of my favorite recipes for Quinoa:

Plum Quinoa Salad

Preparation 20 minutes, cooking time 12 to 15 minutes, chilling time 1 ½ hours.

   1¼ cups quinoa
   2 ½ cups water
   2 large ripe plums, pitted and diced
   ½ cup chopped, toasted walnuts
   ¼ cup chopped red bell pepper
   ¼ cup chopped yellow bell pepper

¼ cup sliced green onions
3 tablespoons flax oil
3 tablespoons extra-virgin olive oil
¼ cup white wine vinegar
1 ½ tablespoon of stevia or natural cane sugar
¼ teaspoon sea salt

Rinse quinoa and drain well. Add to boiling water; reduce heat and sim
mer covered for 12 minutes. Remove from heat and let stand for 5 minutes. Fluff with fork and let chill for about 30 minutes. Stir together
quinoa, plums, walnuts, peppers and onions in a medium bowl. Whisk
together oils, sugar and salt in a small bowl and pour over salad; toss well
to coat all ingredients with dressing. Cover and chill for 1 hour. Makes
6 servings.

Nutrition information per serving; 370 cal., 23g fat (2g saturated), 0g
chol,100mg sodium, 36g carbohydrates, 4g fiber, 8g protein.

This is such a nutritious salad, and very tasty, too. Plums are rich in antioxidants and contain iron, potassium and Vitamin E; flax seed oil contains essential fatty acids and B vitamins; and walnuts are heart healthy
with high amounts of omega-3 fatty acids.

Sun-dried Tomatoes

These tomatoes contain lycopene which is a photochemical and antioxidant that fights free radicals in the body. Sun dried tomatoes contain 12
times the amount of lycopene compared to a regular tomato. They are
a good fat, low in salt content, calories, fat, and contain no cholesterol.
Sun-dried tomatoes are best when mixed with olive oil. They can be used
in salads, chicken dishes, and eggplant or pasta dishes.

Sardines

The name comes from Sardinia, a small island off the coast of Italy.
Sardines contain high levels of Omega-3's which assist in lowering triglyceride levels. Sardines are a great anti-inflammatory. They also are high
in vitamin D, calcium, B12, selenium, protein, and contain three times
the amount of phosphorous than milk, spinach and bananas. They also
contain Coenzyme Q10 (CoQ10), a nutrient found in cells which has

antioxidant and immune system properties. I buy wild sardines in olive oil. I eat them plain or mixed into salads.

Greens

All foods and supplements give off an electrical charge; fresh green live food contains higher frequencies than cooked, processed foods. Dr. Bircher-Benner, a scientific researcher, states "The absorption and organization of sunlight, the essence of life, is derived almost exclusively through plants. Since light is the driving force of every cell in our bodies, that is why we need green plants."

Robert O. Young, Ph.D., a world-renowned microbiologist and nutritionist, heads up the InnerLight Biological Research Center in California. His research in the last 20 years has led to a new biology of eating which includes green alkaline foods.

Green food includes grasses and greens; key ingredients being organic wheat grass, barley, and kamut grass. Irish moss helps to bind mycotoxins and flush them out of the body. Green powder is also an excellent source of protein. Drinking two to three liters a day of green food mixed with pure filtered water also serves as your water quota (usually one-half of your body weight in ounces of water). If you weigh 150 lbs., you would take in 75 ounces of water daily. Water intake is vital to maintain healthy, vibrant skin and bathe your blood cells to halt dehydration.

Green foods also assist in shifting our blood cells and tissues from acid to alkaline. Dr. Young's studies have shown that the blood PH level affects every cell in our bodies. As we change from acid to alkaline, disease cannot exist, weight normalizes, depression lifts, and our quality of life is greatly enhanced. The goal here is to consume 80% alkaline foods or beverages. It's simple to check your acid-alkaline levels using PH strips available at pharmacies. The ideal blood PH is 7.365. Testing first thing in the morning is best.

I had considered my diet healthy until I changed to Dr. Young's suggested food groups while in my 50s. I discovered, for instance, that my breakfast of fruit and yogurt was on the acid side. I started drinking two 32 oz. bottles of green drink daily for a couple of weeks and gradually increased it to three to four 32 oz. bottles. I noticed almost immediately that my joints began to ache as my body gradually released the acid buildup. For me, it began with my feet and traveled up my body to my head.

Juicing

It is difficult to eat four to five servings of vegetables and fruit in one's daily diet. Juice provides a complete compliment of vitamins, minerals and enzymes which nourish your body and improve your health. Drinking two glasses of fresh juice daily along with a balanced diet can give you boundless energy and sometimes reverse long-term illnesses.

I have two juicers; a Vitamix® and a Juiceman®. The Vitamix is pricey but practical. It doubles as a blender to make smoothies and soups as well as juicing vegetables and fruits.

Because I live in the mountains, I tend to eat more warming foods during the winter months; however, come early spring I begin to reintroduce raw foods and juice back into my daily diet. Explore the numerous juicers available and you will discover it is a worthwhile kitchen appliance which serves you well. I encourage you to use fresh farm grown organic ingredients. Juicing will provide fiber to keep you regular and help prevent colorectal cancer. Do not take the easy road by purchasing bottled juices. Often they have preservatives and are heated for pasteurization. They're definitely not fresh so any nutrients are lost. Keep in mind not to juice apple seeds, remove skins from grapefruits and oranges, and eliminate the greens from carrots as they can be toxic.

Cleansing Power Drinks

Today, I make a blended drink with rice or soy milk, protein powder, super greens, avocado, liquid lecithin, and Udo's Choice® Oil Blend, which contains Omega3-6-9 essential fatty acids. Upon rising, I drink a glass of warm water with a squeeze of lemon or lime juice and sometimes I add a pinch of cayenne pepper. This combination balances the PH, provides excellent energy, and is a great morning cleanser.

Drink Your Greens

- Lowers blood pressure
- Improves skin, hair and nails
- Prevents arthritis
- Improves eczema
- Increases metabolic rate to help with weight loss
- Normalizes fat metabolism which may decrease insulin dependency
- Kills cancer cells

Green Tea

There are a variety of different green teas available in the market; Genmaicha is a Japanese tea which is a favorite among adults as well as children. Bancha contains calcium, vitamin A, niacin, and iron. There are many Chinese green teas. I always brew my green tea with care. I do not pour boiling water on the tea leaves and only brew for two to three minutes. A longer steeping period will make the tea bitter tasting.

- Helps retard tooth decay because of its natural fluoride
- Helps with gastrointestinal disorders
- Eases hemorrhoids
- Lowers high blood pressure
- Lowers fever
- Promotes urination
- Eases headaches
- Helps control dizziness
- Dilates blood vessels
- Helps prevent blood clots
- Reduces cholesterol
- Is a powerful anti-oxidant as well!
- Burns calories and helps with weight loss

I also recommend white, black and herbal teas.

What to Avoid (or Minimize)

Before I sound like a preacher, I want to remind you that life is meant to be enjoyed. I am not suggesting you stop eating everything you enjoy, but am asking you to take a look at how often and how much you are eating certain foods and beverages that may be detrimental to your health and well-being over a period of time. Balance, after all, plays a vital role in our day-to-day world.

Corn Syrup

I challenge you to find a traditional food or beverage product that doesn't contain high fructose corn syrup. In a study published in January, 2009 in the *Scientific Journal Environmental Health*, mercury was found in nearly 50% of tested samples of commercial high fructose corn syrup. The news is disturbing given that this ingredient is present in a large portion of processed American foods. According to David Wallinga, M.D., co-author of the study, "Given how much high fructose corn syrup is consumed by children, it could be a significant additional source of mercury never before considered. We are calling for immediate changes by industry and the FDA to help stop this avoidable mercury contamination of the food supply." A separate study by the Institute for Agriculture and Trade Policy detected mercury in nearly one-third of 55 popular brand-name food and beverage products where high fructose corn syrup is the first or second highest labeled ingredient; including products by Quaker®, Hershey's®, Kraft® and Smuckers®.

Sugar

Sugar consumption in the U.S. in 2003 averaged 120 lbs. per person per year. Americans typically use 20 teaspoons of sugar per day. Cutting that consumption in half would help to eliminate excess sugar in our diets. Prior to the turn of the last century (1887 1890), the average sugar consumption was only five lbs. per person per year. Cardiovascular disease and cancer were virtually unknown in the early 1900's; do you think there is a connection? Sugar has been shown to cause inflammation in our bodies, and also attaches to collagen, resulting in stiff, inflexible, sagging skin and is the most aging food for your body and skin. Controlling our blood sugar level and insulin levels will not only improve our overall health, but give us beautiful, youthful skin.

Sugar can lead to an overgrowth of yeast in our stomachs. If you have been diagnosed with Candida, your practitioner will suggest a simple diet without the sugar. Eat several small meals a day and include protein to assist in diminishing your sweet cravings.

Sugar's Side Effects Include:

- Suppressed immune system
- Hypoglycemia
- Coronary heart disease
- Periodontal disease

- Speeds the aging process, causing wrinkles
- Weight gain and obesity
- Depression.
- Kidney damage
- High triglycerides
- High-density cholesterol (HDLs)
- Depletes minerals
- Osteoporosis
- Increases blood platelet adhesiveness, which may result in blood clots and stroke
- Headaches and migraines

Sugar the Natural Way

The FDA has approved Xylitol® (zy-leh-tal) as a sweetener; it is derived from birch—it is not fructose. The World Health Organization has evaluated such Xylitol products as gum, toothpaste, and candies that may prevent tooth decay. It may also help with periodontal disease and strengthen tooth enamel. Xylitol® products are available at your local grocery and health food stores.

Stevia ®(Asteraceae) is a member of the sunflower family. It is also labeled in the marketplace as Sweetleaf®. Stevia® contains certain nutrients, and can be used by diabetics as it does not contain blood glucose.

Carbohydrates

Carbohydrates, protein and fats make up the macronutrients in our diets that provide all our calories. Carbohydrates provide most of the energy needed in our daily lives, both for normal body functions such as heartbeat, breathing, digestion, and for exercise such as cycling, walking and running.

Many people are confused about the differences between simple and complex carbohydrates, and many popular diet books seem to make it more confusing. Carbohydrates are simple or complex based upon their chemical structure. Both types contain four calories per gram. Both are digested into blood sugars called glucose, which is then used to fuel our bodies for work or exercise. The difference is simple carbohydrates are digested quickly. Many simple carbohydrates contain refined sugars and few essential vitamins and minerals. Examples include fruits, fruit juice, milk, yogurt, honey, molasses and sugar, white flour, breads, pasta, and potatoes.

Complex carbohydrates take longer to digest, but also make a lot of acid when they break down. Thus it is best to limit total carbohydrates to 20% of your diet. Feel free to eat broccoli, asparagus, squash, cauliflower, dark greens, celery, cucumbers, sea vegetables, parsley, peas, onions, cabbage, and red, yellow and green peppers. These vegetables are usually packed with fiber, vitamins and minerals. Go easy, however, on carrots, beets and winter squash as they have high sugar content. Avoid, or limit to 20% of your diet, corn, wheat, and rice. Add more spelt, buckwheat, quinoa and millet. These are high in protein, low in acid, non-mucous forming, and help balance sugar levels in the body.

Chocolate

Not all chocolate bars are created equal. Premium Dagoba® bars (available in health food and gourmet stores) contain only four grams of sugar compared to Hershey's Healthy Special Dark Chocolate® which yields 21 grams—more than five times as much sugar. Check the sugar content on the chocolate you purchase, and remember that dark chocolate contains many more benefits (antioxidants, for one) than milk chocolate. The higher the content is of cocoa, the better. Dark chocolate is a natural anti-depressant.

Caffeine

We are a coffee-drinking world. Whether we are sitting at an Italian café sipping an espresso or enjoying a cup of latte at a coffee shop, the tradition of coffee goes way back. Questions have arisen whether or not caffeine is healthy for you. However, in recent years it has been found that coffee can cause dehydration, insomnia, anxiety, increased blood pressure, increased urination, and even diarrhea. It can also increase the risk of osteoporosis.

Is drinking four or more cups daily beneficial for you? One study involved 83,000 American women in their mid-50s who had never had a stroke, diabetes or heart disease brought surprising results. Two to three cups of coffee lowered the risk of stroke by 19%. Women who were non-smokers who drank four or more cups a day reduced the risk of strokes even more to a whopping 43%. It may be a little known fact that twice as many women die from strokes than breast cancer. People who have high blood pressure, insomnia and other related health issues should always consult with their health practitioner before becoming a coffee aficionado.

I am an occasional coffee drinker, usually organic beans and I enjoy a great cup of espresso. I do suggest, however, if you enjoy coffee, purchase organic beans which have not been sprayed with pesticides. When you brew your coffee, use unbleached filters to avoid chlorine leaching into your coffee. Coffee is still acidic (as are sodas), so you may consider switching to herbal teas or black, green or white teas which are packed with antioxidants. Caffeinated teas contain only 90 mg of caffeine compared to 160 mg in coffee. If caffeine is a problem for you, there are many non-caffeinated teas to choose from. Even if a study originates from a professional peer review journal, common sense and moderation can go a long way.

Saturated Fats

Vegetable oils, when heated, form trans-fatty acids and affect our liver's ability to metabolize properly. Serum cholesterol increases and is deposited on the artery walls. LDL (bad) cholesterol levels rise which could lead to arteriosclerosis, heart disease and diabetes. Some of the oils to avoid are canola, corn, soy, and sunflower. These polyunsaturated oils have been shown to contribute to heart disease and weaken the immune system. Canola oil derivative is rape seed, part of the mustard plant family. Rape seed, or canola oil as it is commonly known, is used as a lubricant, fuel and soap so why would one wish to include it as a food? There are many good oils to cook with and to flavor your salads. Avocado oil has a high heat factor (525 degrees) to cook with. It doesn't burn food as easily as safflower, sunflower and canola which have a heat temperature of 225 degrees.

Here is an example of other oils and their heat factors to consider when cooking.

• Almond Oil 495°F

- Corn Oil 450°F
- Peanut Oil 450°F
- Cottonseed Oil 420°F
- Macadamia Nut Oil 410°F
- Sesame Seed Oil (Light) 410°F
- Olive Oil 410°F
- Grape Seed Oil 400°F
- Walnut Oil 400°F
- Coconut Oil 350 F

Graham Kerr, the Galloping Gourmet®, has forsaken the high-fat meals he prepared on his popular television show. His wife and business partner, Treena, discovered that eating rich foods contributed to their seasickness while sailing 24,000 miles on their 71-foot sailboat. In 1981, Treena suffered a stroke and heart attack. Her cholesterol level was at 350. Today she is healthier and her cholesterol is in a safe range.

While we are on the subject of saturated fats, I recently viewed the documentary *Super Size Me*, directed by Morgan Spurlock and released in May 2004. This film received rave reviews at the Sundance Movie Festival and rightly so. The movie addresses how the fast-food industry promotes unhealthy foods and obesity among young and old alike. It follows Spurlock to McDonald's® where he ate three regular meals a day for one month. He had a physical exam performed by three doctors before, during and after the 30-day period. During the 30 days of his McDonald's® diet, his weight ballooned 30 pounds, his cholesterol count went up 65 points, and his blood pressure went from a normal range to high. After the documentary previewed, McDonald's eliminated their "super size" promotions. Just so you know: McDonald's Chief Executive, Jim Cantalupo, died from a massive heart attack and CEO Charlie Bell underwent cancer surgery. Enough said. Grandparents who are concerned about the fast food their grandchildren consume need to see this movie.

Carbonated Soda

Sodas contain phosphoric acid which interferes with the production of calcium, can create weaker bones, and may lead to osteoporosis. Soda also neutralizes stomach acid which aids in digestion. The sugar content equates to ten teaspoons per drink. Ingredients include caffeine, artificial additives and high calories. Health effects include high blood pressure, cholesterol and weight gain.

More No-No's

- Alcoholic beverages
- *Chlorinated water
- Micro-waved foods
- MSG
- Junk and processed foods
- French fries, unless they are baked and preferably sweet potatoes
- Potato chips: try the organic ones, and watch sodium content and added ingredients
- Fried and grilled foods—gas grills only
- Salt, sea salt ok
- Cured and pickled foods
- Mushrooms (however, certain mushrooms such as maitake and shitake are advocated for cancer prevention and treatment)
- Peanuts; peanuts can cause an allergic reaction, and non-organic peanuts are heavily sprayed and may be susceptible to carcinogenic mold spores; an exception to the peanut rule might be Arrowhead Mills® or other organic peanut butter
- Yeast; a gluten test will determine if you are gluten sensitive; if so, eat gluten-free products

Food Toxins

Fluoride

Even though most Western European countries have banned fluoride altogether, Americans ingest it daily through their public drinking water, toothpaste, dental products, beverages and processed foods. Fluoride has been in the U.S. water supply for over 50 years. The fluoride debate has been going on for many years between the ADA (American Dental Association)—which has strong lobbyists in Washington—and independent scientists who have been researching the effects of fluoride for the last 10 years.

As early as 1950, fluoride was given rousing approval by the U.S. Public Health Service which approved of adding it to American drinking water as it was thought to help in the prevention of cavities. Over 60% of the public water in the U.S. now contains fluoride.

The fluoride which is currently used originates from an industrial grade hexafluorosilicic acid used in air-pollution scrubbing systems of the super phosphate industry. The EPA will not permit this substance to be dumped into the oceans but permits it in our drinking water. Fluoride is as toxic as lead and arsenic and contains small amounts of both elements. Some of the ill effects of ingesting fluoride include:

• Brittle bones and increased risk of fractures
• Compromised tooth enamel
• Higher levels of aluminum and lead in the brain and blood
• Compromised immune system which can cause the body to attack its own tissue which may result in tumor growth acceleration

Avoiding Heavy Metals

We have poisoned and continue to poison our environment with cigarette smoke, automobile exhaust, chemical fertilizers, industrial waste, herbicides and pesticides, to name just a few. Our bodies are in constant battle with these heavy toxins, lowering our immune responses and making us susceptible to illnesses and disease. Mercury, in the form of amalgam (silver) fillings in our mouths, has been linked to multiple sclerosis and other autoimmune diseases.

To battle heavy metal toxins in your body, monitor your intake of certain fish and consider having your amalgams replaced with composite fillings. I chose to have my amalgams removed while in my 40s. A simple test can determine the levels of heavy metals in your body; if they are high, you might want to look into chelation therapy, which can be performed intravenously to remove metals.

There are products on the market that claim to release metals from your body. One product that appears to have studies behind it is Zeolite. For more in-depth information refer to the resources section at the end of this book.

Some fish to avoid:

• High POP's (persistent organic pollutants): Farmed salmon; limit to once a month if pregnant/nursing

• High mercury: Atlantic halibut, king mackerel, oysters (Gulf Coast), pike, sea bass, shark, swordfish, tilefish (golden snapper), tuna (steaks and canned albacore)

• Moderate mercury: Alaskan halibut, black cod, blue (Gulf Coast) crab, cod, Dungeness crab, Eastern oysters, mahi mahi, blue mussels, pollock, and tuna (canned light)

• Low mercury but over-fished: Atlantic cod, Atlantic flounder, Atlantic sole, Chilean sea bass, monkfish, orange roughy, shrimp and snapper; these sea creatures should be avoided for the environment's sake

Mercury

I eat fish twice a week. I have always been aware that some fish contain high levels of mercury, but I didn't know how much. After some online research (see the end of this chapter for some good websites), I discovered that four ounces of yellow fin tuna (Ahi) provides 90% of the maximum weekly limit of mercury. I also found that 12 ounces of crab yields 50% of the maximum weekly mercury levels, but 12 ounces of wild Pacific salmon yields only 10%.

The Chicago Tribune investigated mercury levels in canned fish and discovered that albacore tuna contains three times the mercury level of "chunk light" tuna! However, several types of tuna may be blended together, so read your labels. I eat a tuna product from Wild Planet® which is lowest in mercury and is sustainably caught.

Blue Marlin, caught in the Gulf of Mexico, polluted by toxic metals and chemicals dumped into the Gulf of Mexico, can contain 20 to 30 times the acceptable levels of mercury. And the disastrous 2009 BP Gulf Oil spill dramatically changes the picture on whether or not any fish from that area is safe to eat.

There are fish that are lower in mercury and safer to eat, including anchovies, Arctic char, crawfish, Pacific flounder, herring, king crab, sand dabs, scallops, Pacific sole, farmed tilapia, wild Alaska and Pacific salmon; farmed catfish, clams, striped bass, and sturgeon. Wild Alaska and

California salmon (fresh or canned) are also low in Persistent Organic Pollutants (POPs).

Dioxins

Dr. Edward Fujumoto, Wellness Program Director at Castle Hospital, Kailua, Hawaii, says that heating our foods in plastic containers—especially foods that contain fats—releases dioxin, a poison shown to cause breast cancer. Dr. Fujumoto instead recommends using Corning Ware® and/or glass or ceramic containers to heat food in the microwave. He doesn't recommend microwaving TV dinners, instant ramen soups or anything in a paper container. He also believes plastic wraps are dangerous when covered over food heated in the microwave.

Since Dr. Fujumoto's research came out, however, there have been reports that his claims about the release of dioxins are incorrect. The information cited on the internet states that plastic wraps and containers do not contain the chemical components that can form dioxins. Also, this site says that in order for dioxins to be released, temperatures would have to be above 700 degrees Fahrenheit.

My personal view on this controversy is to weigh on the safe side, I will continue using glass containers as advised by Dr. Fujumoto and do further research on this subject. Until proven otherwise, I recommend:

- Do not use plastic containers or plastic wrap in microwave
- Do not put your water bottles in the freezer
- Cover foods in the microwave with glass, ceramic, a paper towel, or parchment paper

Pesticides

Dr. Andrew Weil has stated that environmental toxins can create diseases. However, manufacturers of pesticides have told us that there is no conclusive evidence that there is any harm in eating produce and fruits which have been sprayed with pesticides. What are we to believe? We know that long-term exposure to pesticides can affect the endocrine, hormone, immune, and nervous systems. Pesticides have also been linked to cancer, reproductive problems, and neurological disorders and can be especially harmful to the elderly and anyone suffering from a deficient immune system.

I buy organic produce whenever I can, and wash my fruits and vegetables with a vegetable and fruit wash which can be purchased at any grocery store. Many fruits and vegetables (grapes, apples, cucumbers, etc.) are coated with a wax, so you'll need to scrub all that off. There are a variety of produce washes in the market such as Veggie Wash® which claims it safely and effectively removes wax, soil and agricultural chemicals found on standard and organic produce.

Artificial Sweeteners

Two professors at Purdue University have discovered that artificial sweeteners block the part of you that senses when you're getting full. In other words, they disarm your body's first defense against obesity. Their results, published in the International Journal of Obesity, showed that "mouth feel" plays a crucial role in the body's ability to sense the number of calories that are being consumed—and that artificial sweeteners disrupt the natural calorie "count" based on sweetness.

There are several artificial sweeteners in the marketplace.

• Splenda® is also known as sucralose which is the newest artificial sweetener to hit the market place. It is 600 times sweeter than regular sucrose (table sugar) and converts from cane sugar to a no calorie chemical sweetener. Chlorine is one of the most dangerous chemicals in sucralose. Side effects can include hives, nausea, diarrhea, palpitations and depression. Most short-term studies have been done on animals, with few human studies conducted.

• Aspartame was approved by the Food and Drug Administration in 1981. It is now included in 6,000 food products. It goes by several trade names: NutraSweet®, Equal® and Sugar Twin®. The studies done on the side effects of aspartame have been conflictive. H.J. Roberts, M.D has written a book citing the side effects of ingesting aspartame. Some of these side effects are headaches, abdominal pain, dizziness, anxiety, tinnitus and vomiting.

• Saccharin is the oldest member of the family. It has been available for 100 years. It is known as Sweet and Low®, Sweet N Low®, Sweet Twin®, and Necta Sweet®. A study done in 1977 showed bladder tumors in rats after ingesting saccharin. Rather than removing the product from production and sale, a warning was placed on the product. There were over 30 more studies done and in 2000, National Institute of Health Toxicology Program determined that the 1977 study had high dosages of saccharine and more recent studies showed saccharine to be safe and free of carcinogens. People who have allergic reactions to sulfa may experience dizziness, headaches, diarrhea and shortness of breath.

Due to conflicting studies and reports, it is advisable to research studies on ingesting artificial sweeteners and consider alternatives such as stevia.

Sulfites

I am a label reader, and have been for many years. When my children were small, we would go food shopping together to get them in the habit of reading labels on boxes, cans and frozen foods. One ingredient which appeared over and over was "sulfites." Sulfites appear on labels as sulfur dioxide, potassium bisulfite or potassium metabisulfite, sodium sulfite, sodium bisulfite and sodium metabisulfite. Sulfites supposedly act as a preservative, decrease bacteria growth, and provide longer shelf life—all beneficial to the food industry. However, it's safe to eat products that don't contain sulfites; if you suffer from migraine headaches and food sensitivities, you may want to consider avoiding them.

Some foods that commonly contain sulfites are wine (both red and white), beer, shrimp (fresh and frozen), canned vegetables and fruit, dried fruit, trail mix, potato chips, molasses, condiments, pickled foods and vegetable juices. Also, bacon and ham and processed meats contain sulfites. Who knew so many products contain sulfites. Read the labels in your health food store and grocery store to find products that are sulfite-free.

MSG

Have you noticed that some Chinese menus say "we will omit MSG upon request"? What exactly is MSG (monosodium glutamate)? It is a chemical that seems to be in everything: canned soups, chips, ramen noodles, boxed hamburger mixes, canned gravy, many frozen prepared meals and salad dressings, especially the healthy, low fat ones. Don't be fooled by an ingredient called "hydrolyzed vegetable protein," either. That is just another name for monosodium glutamate. Check your labels.

So why could this chemical be so bad for you? Studies have shown that MSG can be addicting, and that foods containing MSG can cause over-eating and obesity. Some people also have an allergic reaction to it. Fast food chains such as Burger King®, McDonald's®, Wendy's®, Taco Bell® and restaurants like TGI Friday's®, Chili's®, Applebee's® and Denny's® use MSG in abundance.

Years back, I would pick up chicken for my family at Kentucky Fried Chicken® and consume the breaded skin like crazy before I even got home. To my disbelief, I now realize that the crust was coated with MSG. I cringe when I hear the latest commercials for KFC® tout that their chicken now is trans-fat free. That may be well and good; however, I question whether it still contains MSG and if their chickens are free-range and fed a healthy diet.

Is MSG a preservative or a vitamin? It may be neither according to John Erb. In his book *The Slow Poisoning of America*, he wrote an expose of the food additive industry in which he states that "MSG is added to food primarily for the addictive effect it has on the human body."

Food and Health Conditions

Age spots

Older people's skin often develops brown spots on the face and hands. Consider exercising several times a week, limiting excess sun exposure and adding a healthy diet. Dandelion tea helps to cleanse the liver and going on a cleansing diet twice a year, in spring and fall help to lighten the spots. Juice or eat carrot, kale, parsley, spinach, green peppers, grapefruit and lemons.

Aging

This book has discussed nutrition, exercise, supplements and reduction of stress as examples that are extremely beneficial to help slow down the aging cycle. When juicing or eating, consider the deep green leafy vegetables such as kale, broccoli and spinach—all excellent sources of vitamin C, E, selenium and beta carotene.

Alzheimer's Disease (Presenile Dementia)

Remember when cooking in aluminum pots was the norm? Now we have a variety of other cooking options which include ceramic and stainless steel. However, there are many products still in the market place which contain unhealthy levels of aluminum. These include deodorants, drink containers, antacids, buffered aspirin, certain toothpaste, shampoo and baking powder. By avoiding aluminum products you can help to halt the buildup of heavy medals in your body which may prevent a future possibility of getting this disease. Eating sulfur-rich foods helps to cleanse your body of heavy metals. Eating sardines and salmon helps to produce coenzyme Q10, an antioxidant which assists in providing more oxygen in your cells. Juice or eat carrot, kale, parsley, spinach, oranges and grapefruit which supply beta carotene, vitamin C and bioflavonoids.

Osteoarthritis (OA)

This degenerative joint disease is typically characterized by the thin layer of cartilage between the joints which gradually erodes and wears away. As the protective layer of cartilage vanishes, the bone beneath becomes pitted and uneven, and the structural integrity of the joint is destroyed. Movement can become extremely painful and, in the worst cases, people who have severe osteoarthritis can no longer take care of themselves on a day-to-day basis. There are five stages of OA. Although there is no specific cause, risk factors can include obesity, age and muscle weakness of the large muscles around the knee. Physical therapy, knee braces and surgery are some treatments to alleviate OA. Beta-carotene is an anti-oxidant which is found in many foods; spinach, kale, romaine lettuce, pumpkin, cantaloupe, peppers, and carrots.

Rheumatoid Arthritis (RA)

Connective tissues and joints in hands and feet may lead to deformities. Juicing wasn't popular in the middle of the 20th century when my mother was ill with rheumatoid arthritis (RA). Looking back on my mother's diet and weight, I have surmised that by eliminating certain foods and adding others, she may have been able to eliminate many of her chronic symptoms which included pain, swelling of her feet and crippling of her hands; and prevention of future diseases which included lupus. My mom ate certain foods that are from the "night shade" family. These include tomatoes, eggplant, peppers, and potatoes; all of which my mother prepared and were served often at our meals. These vegetables are known to inhibit collagen repair to joints and produce inflammation and degeneration. Certain citrus fruits also have similar reactions; grapefruit, lemons, limes and oranges. Foods that contain Omega-3s, fatty fish, fruits, vegetables, grains and legumes may make symptoms less severe. Juice or eat dark leafy vegetables like kale, broccoli, parsley and spinach which provide excellent sources of vitamin C and pantothenic acid. Add olive oil and soy products, Carrots, ginger root and apples increase copper intake. I remember my mom wearing a copper bracelet. Pineapple contains bromelian which helps with digestion while cherries and blueberries are excellent sources of bioflavonoids.

Atherosclerosis

Hardening of the arteries is a condition which affects millions of people worldwide. Diet and exercise play a huge part in prevention. Avoid caffeine, hydrogenated oils and alcohol. Juice or eat kale, spinach, parsley, carrots, ginger root and garlic which are all beneficial for helping to reduce cholesterol and formation of blood clots.

Cataracts

There are many causes of cataracts: a gradual loss of vision, disease, ultra violet light, radiation, injury and aging. Consultation with an ophthalmologist is advised if you suspect or develop cataracts. To help prevent or delay cataracts, the supplement bilberry helps by removing chemicals from the retina of the eye. It is also high in bioflavonoids. Avoid direct exposure to the sun by wearing sunglasses coated with a UVA and UVB lens. Juice or eat parsley, spinach, garlic, broccoli, orange, ginger root, beet greens which are all excellent sources of vitamin B, E, C and Beta carotene.

Diabetes

Eat a high fiber, whole grain diet with oats, barley and beans along with a good assortment of vegetables and protein. Have citrus fruits and berries, nuts, avocados, olive oil, fish, poultry, eggs and reduced fat dairy products. Obtain a list of foods that are low glycemic foods. Avoid saturated fats and eat small frequent meals to keep your weight in a healthy range.

Heart Disease

High cholesterol, Diabetes Type 2, and obesity are conditions that can lead to heart disease. Foods that support a healthy heart include fruits and whole grains, beans, legumes, nuts, vegetables, potatoes, peas, low fat breads, cereal, rice and pasta. These are low in cholesterol and fat. Avoid baked goods and dishes with cream sauces. Avoid deep fried foods, duck, goose, organ meats, cold cuts and saturated fats. Eat six ounces of protein daily. This includes fish twice a week excluding lobster or shrimp. Eat skim or low fat dairy products. Do not eat fats which include butter, ice creams and sour cream. Limit healthy oils in salads and cooking to eight teaspoons a day.

Inflammation

Inflammation is the basis of many age-related diseases such as heart disease, diabetes, breast and prostate cancer, autoimmune disease, asthma, allergies, arthritis, deteriorating mental ability, and wrinkled, sagging skin. Dr. Samuel West, who has studied the lymph system for many years, claims that healthy cells contain just the right amount of fluid around them without creating any fluid pressure. The blood maintains the fluid pressure by means of blood proteins—albumin, globulin and fibrinogen. It enhances normal cell growth and joint mobility. Inflammation occurs any time a cell is damaged through trauma, injury, toxins from bites, waste products from our metabolism, or micro-organisms like parasites, mold and yeast.

The wrong foods—such as sugar, processed foods, charbroiled and bar-bequed foods, pasta, breads, pastries and baked goods—can increase levels of the pro-inflammatory peptides. Eat vegetables, olive and coconut oil, flax, seeds and nuts, and take aloe vera juice.

Macular Degeneration (AMD)

This is the leading cause of blindness in people 55 and older. Women, drug side effects, family members who have been diagnosed with AMD, high blood pressure, smoking and obesity have been linked to AMD. There are over 10 million people in America that have this disease with a projection of millions more diagnosed by 2020. Macular degeneration occurs when the back of the eye has lost the ability to see things in detail. This makes it difficult to drive, distinguish colors or faces or be able to read. Your sight may be strengthened by eating the Mediterranean Diet which consists of fatty fish high in Omega-3, olive oil, and nuts while avoiding processed high fat foods. Eat leafy green vegetables which contain high amounts of lutein and zeaxanthin. Protect your eyes by wearing sunglasses with UVA and UVB protection, and have periodic eye exams.

Osteoporosis

This disease affects over 75 million people who live in America, Europe and Japan with an expectation of this figure doubling within the next 50 years. Osteoporosis is the most common bone disease leading to low bone mass and deteriorating bone structure. This disease affects more women than men and people with Asian and European ancestry. Osteoporosis increases with age. Hormonal imbalances, inflammation, high blood sugar and significant damage to cell structures (oxidative stress) may contribute to osteoporosis. Fractures are common in the spine, hips and forearms. You can help to maintain strong bones by eating a healthy diet of calcium sources from fruits, green leafy vegetables, beans and yogurt. Limit red meats, caffeine and chocolate. Do weight-bearing exercises as well as brisk walking, aerobics, and tennis. Avoid smoking, excessive drinking, and prescription drugs,

Periodontal Disease

I have a Sonicare® toothbrush. After exploring various brands on the market, I opted to go with one that had good reviews for cleaning teeth and keeping gums healthy. My mom had to have all her teeth pulled before she was 50 because the arthritis and lupus affected her circulatory system and calcium levels. I wish to keep my teeth as long as possible. Proper brushing, flossing and regular check-ups assist in stopping plaque build-up which prevents gingivitis (gum disease) from forming. Excess sugar consumption, drugs, smoking and poor nutrition are just some of the culprits of periodontal disease. Keep your immune system healthy and eat or juice with kale, parsley, garlic, blueberry, cabbage, spinach, ginger and pineapple. Pineapple and ginger are natural anti-inflammatories. By juicing with any of these vegetables you will be receiving the benefits of vitamin C, beta-carotene and zinc to assist in tissue healing, strengthening the immune system, strengthening your heart and reducing gingivitis.

Prostate

Stress and a decrease in male hormone activity may be some of the causes in prostatic hypertrophy. Add higher zinc foods like pumpkin seeds, pecans, whole grains and lima beans. Eliminate beer which increases prolactin, a pituitary hormone. Reducing serum cholesterol levels also helps to prevent prostate problems and inhibit tumor growth. Juice or cook with ginger, parsley, and carrots, all excellent sources of zinc. Kale and spinach elevate vitamin B6.

Shingles (Herpes Zoster)

The same virus that creates chicken pox remains in our nerve cells for years. After age 50, one in five people will get shingles. Shingles can manifest if you are under stress, older, and have a weakened immune system. It can start as a rash on different parts of the body and then become a searing pain which can last for weeks or months depending on the severity of the attack. Help to keep your immune system elevated by eating healthy foods and removing stress from your daily life. A doctor can administer a shot which will help to fight the virus. There is no cure however.

The Dirty Dozen

Based on 2003 USDA figures, a non-profit advocacy group, the Environmental Working Group has listed the top 12 most contaminated fruits and vegetables:

Ranked most contaminated (in order of degree of contamination):

- Peach
- Apple
- Bell pepper
- Celery
- Nectarines
- Strawberries
- Cherries

- Kale
- Lettuce
- Grapes (imported)
- Carrot
- Pear

Least contaminated (in order of least to most):

- Onion
- Avocado
- Sweet corn
- Pineapple
- Mango
- Asparagus
- Sweet peas
- Kiwi
- Cabbage
- Eggplant
- Papaya
- Watermelon
- Broccoli
- Tomato
- Sweet Potato

Though I usually purchase certified organic, some non-organic produce is OK if carefully washed as we've discussed.

Eating in Balance

The key here is creating a balance between our foods; eating less meat and poultry, more vegetables, and less acidic protein in fish and grains. The benefits of dairy products, a source of protein, must be balanced with the drawbacks. Whey, a dairy by-product, is the basis of many protein powders. It can make your blood "dirty" while elevating the white blood cell count. Animal by-products such as cheese, milk and butter, can present a problem, especially if you are lactose intolerant. We believe that we must have milk and dairy in our diets to get the calcium they provide. However, an article in Newsweek stated that the people of Singapore consume almost no dairy and have a much lower rate of osteoporosis than the European countries that consume large amounts of dairy.

Healthy blood builds healthy flesh, bone and muscle. We can help build our blood by consuming 60 grams of polyunsaturated fat a day, such as Omega-3 and Omega-6 oils, vegetable oils, seeds and nuts, flaxseed, and soybean. Greens and essential fats build healthy bodies. The plants we consume produce chlorophyll which is vital for the body's rapid assimilation of amino acids. Its molecular structure is close to hemoglobin which helps to increase oxygen in our system. Chlorella, a derivative from chlorophyll, is noted for improving digestion, eliminating excess mercury, balancing the body's PH, and it adds good bacteria into the intestinal tract, which helps eliminate constipation.

Re-educate yourself on a variety of healthy, nutritious foods, and eat in this new way for the rest of your life. If you consume live, healthy foods and begin and continue a sensible exercise program, your vitality will increase while you are supporting your body's many vital functions. I was recently in a store where two overweight, middle-aged women were discussing how they loved to eat their sweets and why should they deprive themselves of this pleasure? Ask yourself, "Would I rather eat healthy and live healthy for the rest of my life or overindulge and be sick for the rest of my life?" As my grandmother said, "When you have your health, you have everything." The choice is yours.

— Step 4 —

Supplements:
When (Good) Food
is Not Enough

My Story

I gradually began to include vitamin and mineral supplements in my 30s and became more of an advocate of supplements into my 40s. My hormones were changing and the daily demands of being a mother of five children, and a working woman, required more support for my body. Throughout the years I have continually researched new products to assist along my path to wholeness and wellness. For a number of reasons, I find it vital to add supplements to my daily. Upon rising I take the following.

Collagen I and III

Helps support hair, skin, eyes, blood vessels, nails, ligaments, tendons, bones, muscles and weight control.

N-Acetyl Cysteine 600mg

Beneficial amino acid which supports liver functions, helps ward off viruses and assists with chronic lung disorders.

Acetyl L-Carnitine 500 mg

An amino acid which helps convert fat into fuel. It benefits the brain, memory and mood.

Glutathione 500 mg

Considered a first-class free radical scavenger and has the ability to discard carcinogenic chemicals from the body.

Alpha Lipoic Acid 150 mg

Antioxidant which helps to support people who are diabetic, and supports the body against degenerative diseases of the nervous system including Alzheimer's, Lou Gehrig's Disease (ALS) and Parkinson's.

Serrapeptase 40,000 units

Derived from the silkworm, originally discovered in Japan, and used for over 20 years in Europe. Helps reduce inflammation, arterial plaque, clots and scar tissue.

Liquid Chlorophyll

Suggested dosage is one tablespoon in six ounces of filtered water in the morning and before bedtime. The dark greenish color is derived from the cell plant leaves which helps to regenerate bodies at the cellular level, fights infection, heals wounds and detoxifies the body.

I have shortened the list of supplements I consume daily, though at times I may take specific herbs or vitamins depending on my body's current requirements. I look for brands that carry higher amounts of A, B,C,D,E, flax, calcium, magnesium, selenium, chromium, amino acids, herbs, Omega-3 complex and CoQ-10. I currently take a multiple vitamin and mineral formula from a company called Garden of Life® whose products are herbal and raw-food based. I constantly research as new products are always coming into the market, and I will try another line if I am pleased with the company's reputation.

I also take a digestive enzyme with cooked foods. At bedtime, I drink a magnesium and calcium drink along with a capsule of melatonin for sound sleep. When I travel, I carry labeled vitamin boxes.

This is my current program. Everyone has their own personal needs depending on age, health and activity. I highly suggest you tap into your own personal supplement support. I am a bargain shopper and have researched where to buy quality supplements that offer deeper discounts.

Supplements and Health: The Benefits

With today's agriculture methods, we can no longer be sure we are receiving the nutrients necessary for our optimum health. Our soil is often depleted, mass food production is not always of the best quality and Genetically Modified Foods (GMO'S) are becoming more and more prevalent in the food industry. Our diets are just not as wholesome as they were in our grandparents' day. Though they may have consumed large quantities of dairy, meat, eggs, and other foods that were home grown or produced by their neighbor, they contained few food additives and preservatives which today are "required" to preserve freshness or color.

If you eat a moderate amount of fast or processed foods and also have a high level of stress in your life, you definitely will want to consider consulting with your physician/naturopath about adding supplements to your diet.

Synthetic Supplements

- Laboratory conditions may block the production of natural vitamins
- May contain food dyes which can block absorption of B complex vitamins
- Do not contain high levels of antioxidants
- May be made under high heat conditions which over time can produce toxins into the body

Natural Food Base Supplements

- Provide a full complement of fruits and vegetables which the normal person doesn't consume on a daily basis.
- They do not contain chemicals
- Since these are food-based, do your homework on various companies to research the quality of the food source
- Remember to educate yourself on supplement ingredients

Daily Supplements: The Basics

Multi-Vitamin / Mineral Complex

Functions and Uses

Many people take a multi-vitamin/mineral complex every day. They commonly contain thirteen of the essential vitamins, the complete B complex and vital minerals. There are multi supplements that are geared for pregnant women, men and women over 50, and people whose poor nutritional habits need assistance and more nourishment in receiving certain nutrients. Minerals help our cells grow and stay healthy as well as working in synergy with other minerals and vitamins to support vital body functions.

Dosages

Dosages may vary depending on the measurement of ingredients. The Recommended Dietary Allowance (RDA) does not always support certain needs, thus higher strengths may be necessary.

Health Benefits

Vegetarians, as well as people who participate in excessive exercise or experience high stress, benefit by receiving more nutrients.. If you eat a consistent diet of cooked and processed foods, you can also benefit by taking a daily supplement. If you do not take supplements, you can receive multiple benefits by taking an all-around supplement; however be sure you select one of high quality.

Vitamin B Complex

There are eight components that make up this water-soluble complex, each having its own specialized functions for the body. One can take a B complex which would include the following components:

| **Water Soluble Vitamins** |
| Water soluble means that the pill dissolves in water and is not stored in the liver or fat. |

B-1 Thiamine

Functions and Uses

Thiamine supports the heart, muscles and nervous system and helps to convert carbohydrates into energy. People who are thiamine deficient can experience leg cramps, muscle weakness and swelling of the heart. A recent study by the researchers at the University of Warwick in the UK has revealed that high doses of Vitamin B1 or thiamine can also reverse early diabetic kidney disease. Diabetes is the most frequent cause of kidney failure, accounting for nearly 45% of new cases in America alone. Patients with type 2 diabetes, once known as non-insulin-dependent diabetes or adult-onset diabetes, are at much greater risk of developing kidney disease. The onset of kidney disease can be evaluated by a high excretion rate of the protein albumin from the body in the urine through the process known as microalbuminuria; the study at the University of Warwick confirmed that patients taking thiamine for three months showed marked lessening of albumin in the urine.

Dosage

A normal dose is 1.8 mg to 3 mg. Larger amounts have been known to cause toxicity.

B-1 Health Benefits

- Better digestion
- Improved mental ability
- Aids in reducing stress and depression
- Thiamine is found in wheat germ, eggs, leafy green vegetables, legumes, nuts and enriched cereals

B-2 Riboflavin

Functions and Uses

It requires the body to use oxygen and metabolize fatty acids, carbohydrates and amino acids. Deficiencies may show up as sores around the mouth, inflamed tongue, eye disorders, light sensitivity, dizziness, hair lose and insomnia.

Dosage

The average dosage is 50 mg per day along with 50 mg of B-6. For better absorption, take with vitamin C. Higher amounts can be taken if on a weight loss diet, under stress, drink alcohol, or taking antibiotics.

B-2 Health Benefits

• Healthier skin, hair and nails
• Increases energy in the body
• Supports healthy red blood cells
• Provides antioxidants to help slow down aging
• Foods that are high in B-2 are yogurt, fish, green leafy vegetables, dairy, nuts and grains

B-3 Niacin ~ Nicotinic Acid ~ Vitamin P or Vitamin PP

Functions and Uses

It is found in plants and animal tissues. In 1915, Dr Joseph Goldberger discovered a link between prison inmates fed low amounts of niacin through their diet. He coined the word "pellagra" (the disease of the four Ds: dementia, diarrhea, dermatitis and death). By adding niacin rich foods Dr. Goldberg was able to reverse the inmates' symptoms.

B Vitamin Rich Foods

Foods that have B vitamin benefits include green vegetables, whole grains, lentils, potatoes, bananas, dairy products, eggs, turkey liver, and tuna. Take B complex earlier in the day. Taking B complex later may interrupt a sound sleep.

Dosage

The suggested RDA is 19 mg for males and 13 mg for females per day. Too little produces mental confusion, irritability and diarrhea. Alcoholism can make people deficient in B-3. Harmless flushing of the skin may occur, but if a medical condition arises, it is advisable to consult with your practitioner about taking higher dosages.

B-3 Health Benefits

• Supports the nervous system, sex hormones, skin, stomach, intestinal tract and removes toxins

- It helps reduce bad cholesterol (LDL) and increases good cholesterol (HDL) and promotes better circulation
- It helps people with osteoarthritis, rheumatoid arthritis and insulin-dependent diabetes
- Food sources include salmon, tuna, chicken, peas, dried beans, sunflower seeds, beets, brewer's yeast, veal, pork and turkey

Pantothenic Acid B-5

Functions and Uses

B-5 plays a role in metabolizing fats, carbohydrates and proteins. Pantothenic acid is an essential nutrient to sustain life. People take B-5 for dietary deficiencies to treat respiratory disorders, lower blood sugar, carpal tunnel syndrome, depression, fatigue, celiac disease, headaches, asthma, osteo- and rheumatoid arthritis, Parkinson's disease, shingles, enlarged prostate and multiple sclerosis. It also helps produce vitamin D.

Dosage

The average dosage is 5 mg although people may take up to 250 mg a day. Too much pantothenic acid can produce anxiety and over stimulation and may lead to diarrhea.

B-5 Health Benefits

- People experience more vitality
- Better moods
- Alertness
- Wound healing
- Food sources include yogurt, avocados, peas, beans, poultry and organ meats

B-6 Pyridoxine

The blood and nervous system require B-6 to function well. It converts tryptophan (amino acid) to niacin. B-6 makes hemoglobin, which carries oxygen to tissues. B-6 deficiency can make one iron deficient and anemic. Other symptoms caused by B-6 deficiency include dermatitis, confusion and depression.

Dosage

The RDA recommendation for people over age 50 is 1.5 mg for women, 1.7 mg for men. For adults, it is considered safe to take from 50 to 100 mg per day. When taken in high doses (200 mg or more per day) over a long period of time, vitamin B-6 can cause neurological disorders such as loss of sensation in legs and imbalance. Symptoms are reversed when that dosage is no longer taken.

B-6 Health Benefits

- Balances estrogen and progesterone levels
- Acts as a diuretic
- Formation of red blood cells
- Regulates blood pressure
- Improves the nervous system
- Food sources high in B-6 include calve's liver, sardines, snapper, shrimp, halibut, Chinook salmon, lamb, beef tenderloin, and venison

Vitamin B-12 Cobalamin

Functions and Uses

This is the most complex of the B vitamins. A vegetarian diet is more likely to be deficient in B-12 than one which includes meat, fish, eggs and milk. Deficiencies in B-12 may also be caused by malabsorption which can lead to pernicious anemia. Pernicious anemia destroys Intrinsic Factor (IF), an enzyme secreted by the stomach necessary to produce B-12. B-12 deficiency may cause dementia which is closely correlated to the early stages of Alzheimer's disease (AD). Lower levels of B-12 may elevate homocysteine (amino acid) which may lead to heart disease. Depression, memory problems and nervousness also may be signs of a deficiency. Taking B-12 in conjunction with folic acid and B complex helps improve healthy heart functions.

Dosage

Absorption of B-12 can decrease with age. B-12 is stored in small amounts in the body, so daily doses may not be required. The RDA for adults is currently 2.4 mcg per day, but can range as high as 3,000 mcg daily. According to the Institute of Medicine of the National Academy of Sciences, there are no adverse effects from large doses of Vitamin B-12. People with eating disorders and inflammatory stomach and intestinal disorders may require higher dosages, as their ingestion of B-12 can be slowed. B-12 also can be absorbed through a skin patch, injection, or sublingual tablet. If you question your B-12 levels, there are numerous tests to evaluate whether you are low in this B vitamin. It is impossible for the body to store too much B-12.

B-12 Health Benefit

• Healthy nervous system
• Better digestion
• Carbohydrate metabolism
• More energy
• Sharper memory
• Fewer migraines
• Improved skin, nails and hair
• Food sources high in B-12 include shell fish, lamb and beef liver, mackerel, herring salmon, tuna, beef, cheese, and eggs

Folic Acid ~ Folate ~ Folinic Acid

Functions and Uses

Folic acid manufactures red blood cells and a lack of it may cause anemia. It lowers homocysteine (amino acid) levels to help improve heart health. High levels of homocysteine have been connected to Alzheimer's disease, strokes and osteoporosis. Low levels of folic acid have been linked to alcoholism, liver disease, colon and cervical cancer. Pregnant women need to take folic acid to prevent spina bifida (spine and back mis-development) in the fetus. People who are on kidney dialysis can also benefit by taking folic acid.

Dosage

A normal dose is 400 mcg per day. During the early stages of pregnancy, the recommended dosage is 400 to 800 mcg per day. If you have health issues, consult with your practitioner regarding how much folic acid you should take.

Folic Acid Health Benefits

- Strengthens fragile bones (osteoporosis)
- Lifts depression
- Helps improve macular degeneration (eye disease)
- Wards off hearing loss
- Improves memory
- Deters Alzheimer's disease

B-7 Biotin ~ Vitamin H

Functions and Uses

Biotin research began in the early 1900's. The research went on for 40 years before it was acknowledged as a vitamin. Biotin is important in cell growth as well as metabolizing fats and amino acids. It helps the body to use glucose (blood sugar) for body fluids. Deficiencies include hair loss, rash around the mouth, eyes and nose, tingling in the arms and legs, depression, brittle nails and thinning hair. Biotin has been coined the "beauty vitamin" and is included in many hair and nail products.

B Vitamin Dosages

Before taking a B complex supplement, you might want to consult your health care provider. People's bodies vary, and while some may require a higher dosage of B-12, for example, others would benefit from a higher ratio of another of the B vitamins.

Dosage

The suggested dosage is 30 to 100 mcg daily. Higher amounts up to 2,500 mcg have been safe to take. Diabetics have taken 5 to 1.5 mg to help reduce their blood sugar.

B7 Health Benefits

- Strengthens hair and nails
- Good for weight loss
- Biotin combined with chromium may help reduce blood sugar in

diabetics

- Foods which contain biotin are egg yolks, brewer's yeast, wheat germ, molasses, peanuts and peanut butter, oatmeal, beans and legumes, fish, breads, poultry, cauliflower, mushrooms, dairy products and bananas

Vitamin C ~ Ascorbic Acid

Functions and Uses

This supplement is a water soluble antioxidant nutrient which helps block free radicals from building up which create aging in the body. Deficiencies in vitamin C can cause bleeding gums, bruising, decrease in the body's ability to fight infections, painful and swollen joints and rough skin.

Linus Pauling was a renowned scientist and winner of the Nobel Peace Prize. This remarkable man was a strong advocate of taking increasingly higher dosages of vitamin C to ward off diseases and the common cold. He coined the term "orthomolecular" meaning the right molecules in the right amount. His research on vitamin C has been highly debated throughout the years. He died at the age of 94.

Foods High in Vitamin C

Food sources of vitamin C are broccoli, brussel sprouts, cabbage, cauliflower, red peppers, winter squash, leafy greens, raspberries, cranberries, blueberries and pineapple.

Dosage

Suggested dose is 2,000 mg daily or lower. Some side effects of higher amounts may include diarrhea and stomach upset. Vitamin C comes in powder and pill variety. I prefer the powder added to water, juice or into a protein drink.

Vitamin C Health Benefits

- Vitamin C helps heal wounds
- Builds stronger bones, cartilage and teeth
- As an antioxidant, vitamin C helps fight off diseases like cancer, heart disease, and inflammatory conditions such as arthritis

Vitamin D

Functions and Uses

As children we were told to drink our milk for our bone health because that, along with diet, would supply our daily dose of vitamin D. Medical doctors are now recognizing that vitamin D is playing biologic roles in peoples' health, thanks to Dr. Michael Holick, the world's leading researcher on vitamin D. According to his research, vitamin D appears to play a vital role in cancer prevention as well as cancer treatment. Deficiencies show up as aches, pains and weakness in muscles and bones. Many people are vitamin D deficient compared to our hunter forefathers who were exposed to the sun all day. Because of the rise in skin cancer, it is now recommended that we wear sunscreen protection and do not expose ourselves to the sun between 10:00 a.m. and 2:00 p.m. However, our bodies only produce vitamin D during those hours. The cold winter months contribute to vitamin D deficiency as well. If we are not to be in the sun as our forefathers were, we may need to consider supplementation.

Dosage

Dr. Holick suggests that children need a daily dose of between 400 and 1,000 IU; teenagers and adults between 1,500 and 2,000 IU daily. Since older people produce 75% less vitamin D in the body, Dr Holick recommends that people over the age of 70 have more sun exposure to their backs, legs, arms and abdomen while protecting their face. According to a study done in 2003 with Dr. Robert Heaney of Creighton University Research Center, one can take 10,000 IU of vitamin D daily for six months without toxicity. One can take D with or without food daily, weekly or monthly as long as you receive the recommended dose.

Vitamin D Health Benefits

- Improves mood
- Helps build bone mass
- Prevents autoimmune disease, colds and flu
- May also help to reduce risks of cancer, decrease inflammation and chronic pain

- Helps obese people by stimulating fat cell metabolism
- Stimulates insulin production for diabetics
- Good food sources include dairy products, wild caught salmon, sardines, shrimp, halibut, trout, tofu, soy milk, milk and orange juice

Vitamin E ~ d-Alpha-Tocopherol

Functions and Uses

This is a fat soluble vitamin which can be stored in the body up to six months. It comes in eight different forms with d-alpha-tocopherol being the most active. It also acts as a powerful antioxidant which protects cells against free radicals, therefore helping to protect the body from cancer and cardiovascular diseases that can occur when cells are damaged. Gamma tocopherol is less strong but very essential for maintaining healthy cell membranes, especially when d-alpha-tocopherol is present. A recent study done by Australia's Queensland University of Technology demonstrates that gamma tocopherol has the ability to inhibit prostate cancer stem cells.

Dosage

A recommended amount of 800-1,600mg per day, if not consuming vitamin E from food sources. Otherwise absorption of vitamin A and K can be compromised. Other forms of vitamin E can be taken. The cold water form (alpha tocopherol succinate/acetate) is twice as expensive as the soy-based oil. It is effectively absorbed on an empty stomach if taken with several grams of a fat or oil. A second form is soybean oil (E-acetate) which is low in saturated fat and does not contain cholesterol. Liquid vitamin E absorbs better than the capsule form. Selenium, magnesium and vitamin A will increase the benefits of vitamin E.

Vitamin E Health Benefits

- Reduces cholesterol; lowers chances of stroke and coronary artery disease
- Helps protect eyes
- Protects against UV radiation

- Heals wounds
- Keeps skin moist
- Helps relieve arthritic pain
- Good food sources include wheat germ oil, almonds, sunflower seeds, mustard and turnip greens, and spinach

Vitamin K

Functions and Uses

This fat-soluble supplement was discovered by Edward Adelbert Doisy and Henrik Dam who won a Nobel Peace Prize in 1943. The "K" stands for the German word "koagulation," as it assists in coagulating blood. It also assists in normal bone calcification. Low vitamin K is associated with lower bone density and common hip fractures and often can affect the elderly, Deficiencies show up as bruising and bleeding. People on antibiotics show poor absorption of K in the intestinal tract.

Dosage

If you are on an anticoagulant drug, consult with your physician before taking vitamin K. Consider obtaining a supplement that contains all three of the K forms; MK-7,MK-4 and K1. Although a small amount of K (80mcg) is sufficient for clotting blood, higher dosages are beneficial for age-related diseases and safe to take.

Vitamin K Health Benefits

- Fewer heart attacks
- Increase bone mass in post-menopausal women
- Regulates blood sugar
- Reduces bone fractures especially in post-menopausal women
- Treats heavy menstrual bleeding
- Normal blood clotting
- Good food sources include Brussel's sprouts, spinach, kale, cauliflower, broccoli, cabbage and soybeans

Good to Consider Supplements

Calcium (CA) Calcium Carbonate~ Calcium Citrate ~Calcium Malate

Functions and Uses

This major mineral is primarily stored in the bones and teeth with smaller amounts found in the blood, muscles and extra cellular fluid. At a younger age, the body continues to break calcium down and build it up to help support strong bones. As we age, calcium requirements become higher because the mineral becomes stored in the body more than it's replenished.

Dosage

Dosages may vary depending on age. After age 50 the requirements are at 1,200 mg per day. Taking vitamin D with calcium helps to absorb the calcium into your body. If you take more than 2,500 mg per day it may interfere with other minerals as well as affect healthy kidney functions. If you have certain health conditions such as heart problems, bone tumors or kidney problems, consult your physician to determine if this is a supplement you can take.

Calcium Health Benefits

- Treats osteoporosis
- Helps to build bones
- May help control high blood pressure
- Protects pre-menopausal women against breast cancer
- Calcium is found in milk, cheese, yogurt, sardines, broccoli, kale, and dark green leafy vegetables

Magnesium (MG)

Functions and Uses

Magnesium is a crucial mineral which supports over 300 chemical reactions in the body to have it work efficiently. Our soil is depleted of MG due to the use of fertilizers. Though the normal body contains 25 grams, it is common for women, African Americans, and the elderly to have a magnesium deficiency. Surface water contains very small amounts of MG and certain medicines can also deplete magnesium in the body. Magnesium deficiency may create physical and mental stress and loss of potassium and calcium through urination.

Dosage

Many calcium and magnesium supplements have a ratio of 2:1 calcium to magnesium. For instance, if your supplement contains 1,200 mg of calcium, the magnesium would be 600 mg. If you have a kidney disease or other conditions, consult with your physician before taking.

Magnesium Health Benefits

- Assists in heart regulation
- Healthy bones
- Normal blood pressure
- Helps treat diabetes
- Treats kidney stones
- Relieves asthma
- Helps people with multiple sclerosis
- Reduces migraine headaches
- Helps altitude sickness
- Helps stomach acid

> **Foods High in Magnesium**
>
> Some foods that contain magnesium are broccoli, squash, dark green leafy vegetables, beans, whole grains, chocolate, coffee and almonds.

Coenzyme Q10 ~ CoQ10

Functions and Uses

This fat-soluble vitamin-like compound called ubiquinone plays an important role inside our human cells allowing for healthy cellular growth, energy production, and immune and antioxidant support. The highest amount of CoQ10 is found in the heart. There have been numerous scientific studies done on the benefits of taking CoQ10. Many have to do with heart disease. Unusually low levels of CoQ10 have been reported with people who have high blood pressure.

Dosage

A healthy adult can take between 30-100 mg per day. People who have heart conditions may take dosages of 150 mg per day with a practitioner's consultation. Some studies have linked the diminishing of women's breast tumors after taking 390 mg for one month. CoQ10 assimilates best when taken with a small amount of fat such as peanut butter or olive oil.

CoQ10 Health Benefits

• Prevents fatty acid build up within the heart muscle

• Converts to energy which assists the heart in functioning better

• Helps with high blood pressure

• Helps chronic fatigue

• Weight loss

Essential Fatty Acids ~ EFA's

Functions and Uses

EFA's are found in every cell throughout our body. Omega-3's ALA (alpha linoleic acid) is vital because of its ability to suppress inflammation in the body which helps prevent degenerative diseases such as heart disease, Alzheimer's, rheumatoid arthritis and diabetes. 8% of the brain's weight consists of Omega-3's. This contributes to improved memory, mental health and Alzheimer's prevention. People who are depressed or have attempted or committed suicide have been shown to have reduced levels of DHA and EPA in their red blood cell membranes or serum. Unlike Omega-3, Omega-6 creates inflammation. The healthy ratio between Omega-6 and Omega-3 is a range of 3:1 (3 parts Omega-3 to 1 part Omega-6) or 4:1 (4 parts Omega-3 to 1 part Omega-6).

Dosage

Omega-3's 1,000-3,000 mg of EPA and 1,000-1,500 mg of DHA. One need not take Omega-6 in pill form if Omega-6 food sources are consumed on a daily basis or a pharmaceutical grade of EFA's oil contains a ratio of 3:1 or 4:1.

EFA'S Health Benefits Omega-3

- Anti inflammatory
- Relieves menopause symptoms
- Alleviates depression
- Helps heart, breast and bone health
- Reduces high blood pressure
- Relieves arthritis symptoms
- Reduces high cholesterol
- Reverses early stages of Alzheimer's
- Helps prevent osteoporosis
- Helps prevent obesity
- Helps prevent prostate problems
- Omega-3 food sources include wild salmon, sardines, herring, mackerel, flaxseed, walnuts, pumpkin seeds, eggs, fruits, vegetables and olive oil

Health Benefits Omega-6

- Maintains healthy brain function
- Reduce nerve pain for diabetic neuropathy
- Reduces pain and swelling for rheumatoid arthritic conditions
- Builds strong bones
- Healthy skin
- Helps alleviate hot flashes and night sweats
- Omega-6 food sources are evening primrose oil, borage oil, sunflower oil, olive oil, safflower oil, wheat germ oil, flaxseed oil, sesame oil, hempseed oil, almonds, pistachios, olives, chicken, and turkey

Conjugated Linoleic Acid (CLA)

Functions and Uses

Approximately 34% of the current U.S. population is classified as obese. One billion people worldwide are obese according to the World Health Organization (WHO). Weight escalates during holiday seasons when we all tend to overeat. If CLA can contribute to reducing body fat and slowing or reversing weight gain (according to the International Journal of Obesity and Professor Schoeller), then doesn't it make sense to take CLA along with your sensible nutrition and exercise plan?

CLA helps the body break down and use the fat normally stored after meals. It decreases body fat mass, maintains lean body mass, and aids in weight management—reducing the "yo-yo" effect often associated with diet plans. A study published in late 2005 by the Journal of Nutrition found that adults taking a CLA supplement lost as much as 9% of their body fat. As important, a follow-up 12-month study found that participants did not regain their body fat.

To get three grams of CLA through food alone, an adult would have to consume more than 4 gallons of ice cream or 28 quarter-pound hamburgers every day. Obviously, CLA supplementation is the only way to go. Supplementation with CLA is most effective as part of a daily regimen that includes exercise and a reasonable diet.

Dosage

With each meal, take 1,000 mg of CLA. Tonalin® CLA is derived from natural safflower oil and the company claims it is the most clinically tested CLA on the market. Tonalin® CLA is stimulant-free and is available in health food stores, retail chains and online.

CLA Health Benefits

- Reduces body fat
- Cholesterol metabolism
- Lower triglycerides
- Lowers insulin resistance
- Enhances immune system

Lutein

Functions and Uses

This is a naturally occurring carotenoid which is a natural coloring found in vegetables and fruits. This supplement plays a critical role in support of healthy eyes. It acts as a protection from blue light in indoor lighting as well as sunlight.

Dosage

Take 6 to 10 mg of lutein and 1 mg of zeaxanthin daily. For older people with poor digestion, a sublingual spray is available.

Lutein Health Benefits

- May help reduce cataracts
- May help to reduce risks of age related macular degeneration (AMD)
- May supply antioxidant properties
- Lutein is naturally found in foods which include dark green leafy vegetables, romaine lettuce, pistachio nuts, and egg yolks

Chromium

This is an essential trace mineral which helps to regulate sugar through the cells and reduce glucose levels in the blood. People with Type 1 and Type 2 Mellitus Diabetes may benefit by taking this supplement. Consult with your physician.

Dosage

A suggested dosage is between 50 and 200 mg daily. The side effects are rare at these dosages.

Chromium Health Benefits

- May help control abnormal glucose intolerance in Type 2 Diabetes
- May help to control cholesterol levels
- May help to control fat
- May help reduce cravings for sweets
- Food sources include eggs, brewer's yeast, chicken, potatoes, apples, peas, broccoli, and mushrooms

Alpha Lipoic Acid

This sulfur-containing fatty acid is present in all human cells. In 1988, alpha-lipoic acid was recognized as an effective anti-oxidant which helps to neutralize free radicals that can damage cells. Free radicals contribute to aging and chronic illnesses. It also increases the production of glutathione which helps to dissolve toxic substances from the liver. It may help people with cataracts, glaucoma, multiple sclerosis, Parkinson's and Alzheimer's disease.

Dosage

If you are healthy, dosages are 50-300 mg daily. For people who have diabetes, 100 to 200 mg three times a day is a suggested dosage. Taking dosages higher than 1,800 mg could cause headaches, nausea and low blood sugar.

Alpha-Lipoic Health Benefits

* May help the body utilize insulin more effectively
* May help with inflammation in joints arteries and muscles
* Improves blood flow and circulation to the body and the brain
* Helps to reduce environmental toxins to the cells
* Helps strengthen heart muscles and arteries
* Food sources include peas, broccoli, Brussels sprouts, and spinach

Store supplements in a cupboard away from heat and check expiration dates on the bottle. Some supplements require refrigeration after opening. Educate yourself on brands with a good reputation and look to see if they are synthetic or natural. If in doubt, consult with a physician, naturopath, health food expert or other professional familiar with this topic. If you are under a physician's care for a chronic health problem, consult with your doctor before taking any supplements.

> ### When to Take Supplements
>
> A suggestion is to take amino acids on an empty stomach. For better absorption take fat soluble supplements with foods that contains oil or fat. Take supplements at breakfast and lunch. Herbal sleep aids can be taken an hour before bedtime.

Supplements, Drug Therapies, and Health Conditions

Insomnia

Each person has their own definition of insomnia. 30 to 50% of people have acknowledged having occasional insomnia while 10% are chronic insomniacs. It appears that women are more affected than men. Ageing, excessive drinking, stress, depression and poor mental health can all play a role in our sleeping patterns. Physiological causes range from circadian rhythm disorders to a host of physical conditions including chronic pain, heart problems, sleep apnea, asthma, Parkinson's disease, Alzheimer's disease and disturbances of the brain such as strokes and brain tumors.

Hormones and Sleep

Our bodies normally produce human growth hormone (HGH) which aids in sleep. Our adrenal glands are restored during sleep; but with lack of sleep, cortisol, which is produced through our adrenals, becomes elevated and results in sluggishness, constipation, PMS, bloating and a low libido. By the time we reach fifty, the amount of sleep begins to decline by 27% a decade, and HGH secretion decreases by 78% over this period. Less HGH is produced by the body because of less deep sleep. However, HGH replacement therapy has confirmed that patients taking HGH sleep better. Excess fat in the body can destroy HGH levels.

Supplement Suggestions Before Bedtime

- Melatonin
- Valerian
- DHEA
- Calcium ~ magnesium
- Chamomile tea
- Tryptophan
- 5- HTP

Depression

Over 14 million Americans have been diagnosed with depression. There are a multitude of causes. It could be a loss of a loved one, a loss of a job or home, health conditions, being older or shifts in hormones and medications. Depressed people seem to lose interest in life, become anxious or irritable and may even contemplate suicide.

Supplement Suggestions

- Omega-3 fatty acids
- SAM-e
- Folic acid
- Magnesium
- Tryptophan
- Morpheme Memocare (Ayurvedic)
- Licorice tea
- St John's Wort

Osteoporosis

When my mother slipped in the tub and broke her hip, she had been on steroid medication for an accelerated rheumatoid arthritic condition, and the steroid treatments were not supplemented with any vitamins or minerals. Statistically, there is a 30% mortality rate within the first year after suffering a hip fracture. My mother lived for seven more years, but not without constant pain, swelling and an ambulatory condition which severely compromised her health. She developed lupus and had a stroke in her early 50s.

Osteoporosis causes a loss of bone density, contributing to the 1.5 million fractures (including 300,000 broken hips) suffered annually. Women especially face bone loss during menopause due to reduced estrogen production. Contrary to popular belief, men can also be affected by osteoporosis, but usually five to ten years after women.

My family history showed no indication of rheumatoid arthritis (RA). Observing and living with a parent who experienced constant severe pain was emotionally difficult for family members, however her condition helped me to become more aware of my own wellbeing and thus I became more health minded through my lifetime.

Supplement Suggestions

- Calcium, vitamin D, zinc, copper, magnesium, boron
- Vitamin C, B12, vitamin K, folic acid and silicon are essential for stronger bones

- Trace minerals and magnesium can help support healthy bone function
- Take 1,000 IU of vitamin D, 1,200 milligrams of calcium and 400 milligrams of magnesium

If you wish to research this subject further, refer to the references at the end of the book. This offers a wealth of research as well as advice on supplements and diagnostic testing. In Chapter Three, the Healthy Numbers also provides more information on osteoporosis.

Menopause

My Menopause story

While in my mid-40ss, I began to experience pre-menopausal symptoms which included night sweats, irregular menstrual cycles, poor sleeping patterns and emotional irritations. It wasn't until I almost reached 50 that I was post-menopausal. I was and still remain very physical. I read once that a professional ballet dancer can exhibit irregular hormones and experience cessation of her menstrual cycle at a young age due to their vigorous training, but once they stop their training, their cycle returns to normal. I began my cycle when I was 12 years old so I reasoned that I was approaching post-menopause at an earlier age. I had never gone on birth control, nor was I a pharmaceutical or over-the-counter user, so I visited my Chinese doctor. The doctor prescribed Chinese medicine and gave me a series of acupuncture treatments that helped to lessen some of the symptoms and I rode it out. There weren't any bio-identical testing methods back then and because my preference had always been to go the herbal route, that felt like the best course for me to take.

Hormone Replacement Therapy

Wyeth Pharmaceuticals, manufacturers of Premarin® and Prempro® is asking the FDA to deny Americans access to bio-identical hormone replacement drugs prepared by compounding pharmacies and available only under a doctor's prescription. These custom-made preparations combine individualized doses of hormones chemically identical to those found in the human body. Prescription hormones such as Premarin® are proving to have certain unsafe side effects, leading to more physicians prescribing bio-identical hormone replacement therapies.

Bio-identical formulations can be made without additives and dyes commonly found in conventional, one-size-fits-all prescription drugs. Moreover, the use of compounded hormones allows for specialized, flexible dosing strategies. This is consistent with the most recent FDA Menopause and Fact Sheet (issued in July 2005), which recommends that menopausal hormone therapy should be used at the lowest doses for the shortest duration needed to achieve treatment goals. Hormones decrease dramatically in aging adults, including menopausal women. Lowered hormone production associated with age results in decreased bone mass, hot flashes, diminished libido, vaginal dryness, allergies, fatigue, poor sleep, sugar cravings, excess fat and memory lapses.

Restoring hormones for men and women alike will produce many benefits including relief from depression, insomnia, migraine headaches, low energy, low libido, and mental fatigue.

Get advice from your physician or health care practitioner before starting hormone replacement therapy during and after menopause.

Hormone / Insulin-Cortisol Balance

Refined sugar and starchy foods create an overload of blood sugar and when it hits our cells, blood sugar levels drop. Decreased blood sugar levels create stress in our brains and cortisol kicks in. Stress produces higher levels of cortisol, which in turn depletes progesterone levels. Our bodies use progesterone as a building block to make cortisol, so when we manufacture high levels of cortisol we deplete progesterone and disrupt its balance with estrogen.

Insulin is a hormone that transports blood sugar to our cells to be used as energy. When our body is producing excess amounts of cortisol, overweight individuals can become insulin-resistant, becoming more immune to insulin's effects.

Supplement Suggestions

• Soy isoflavones – 40 mg daily
• Indole-3-Carbinol – 300-500 mg daily

- Chromium – 200-600 mg daily
- DHEA – 10- 25 mg daily; monitor reaction
- L-Carnitine – 500 mg daily
- CoQ10 – 100-200 mg daily
- Red Clover (Trifolium pratense) – helps with hot flashes, contains high levels of isoflavones (estrogen-like plant compounds). 15-30 drops, 3 times daily; do not use with blood-thinning drugs; helps improve cardiovascular health
- Vitex/Chasteberry (vitex agnus-castus) – 30 drops or one cup of tea three times daily; results may be felt after three months; helps regulate progesterone and estrogen levels; calms anxiety, bloating, irritability and depression
- Black Cohosh (Cimicifuga racemosa) – 40 mg daily. Contra-indications: headache, nausea; is an alternative to hormone replacement therapy; helps relieve hot flashes, mood swings and vaginal dryness, improves bone strength, and most importantly, doesn't raise estrogen levels
- B complex – 50-100 mg daily
- Vitamin C/ bioflavonoids – 1,000-2,000 mg daily
- Calcium – 1,200 mg daily
- Magnesium glycinate – 400 mg daily
- Magnesium oxide – 600 mg. (Rule of thumb: magnesium dosage is usually one half of calcium dosage; i.e., 1,200 mg calcium=600 mg of magnesium)
- Fish oil – 5,000 mg daily
- Zinc – 25-50 mg daily

Alzheimer's

This is the most common form of dementia and is the sixth leading cause of death in the U.S. Alzheimer's disease has affected 26 million people worldwide. There have been Alzheimer topics discussed throughout the book which include symptoms, testing, diet, and exercise.

A United States research study has shown that people who take angio-tension-receptor blockers are 35 to 40% less likely to develop Alzheimer's disease. Angiotension-receptor blockers are drugs that are used to lower blood pressure.

In addition to the good news with respect to preventing Alzheimer's disease, the study showed that even if a person already has the illness, starting the angiotension-receptor blockers would slow the progression of the illness down by 45%. Professor Clive Ballard of the Alzheimer's Research Society is quoted as saying, "This study highlights that it is becoming increasingly important to investigate blood-pressure lowering drugs as a potential treatment for dementia."

Supplement Suggestions

• Multiple vitamin/mineral
• Essential fatty acids
• Minerals
• Alpha lipoic acid – 50 mg
• Acetyl L- Carnitine – 300 mg
• Choline – 100- 500 mg
• Curcumin
• Mind Power RX herbal brain formula

Inflammation

Chronic inflammation is rapidly becoming a major factor in diseases and in aging. Poor diet, drugs, stress and toxins all play a role in the formation of inflammation in our bodies. Often inflammation occurs in joints and cartilage for people who have arthritis.

As discussed earlier, testing by bio-chemical markers c-reactive proteins can measure the amount of inflammation in the body. Many of the mainstream pharmaceutical anti-inflammatory drugs carry side effects.

Serrapeptase

Serrapeptase, a derivative of the silkworm has been tested and used in Europe for over ten years with rousing success. This pain relief and anti-inflammatory product is cultivated from silkworms, which use the enzyme to break down the hard shell of their cocoon soon after birth. It has been used in Japan and Europe for over 30 years and is available in prescription form in Austria and Germany. It was introduced into the USA as recently as 2002. German coronary physician Dr. Hans Nieper used serrapeptase to unblock arteries in his heart patients. It dissolved blood clots and caused varicose veins to shrink or diminish. Because it is a natural anti-inflammatory, it can dissolve the dead proteins that bind plaque which can block the arteries, supports normal cell growth, joint function, and cardiovascular function.

I have been taking serrapeptase every day as a preventative measure. A woman I know who is in her 40s began to take one pill a day and noticed her varicose veins fading in a week's time. Serrapeptase is a natural product that can be taken safely both short- and long-term, and will not interfere with other medications. No side effects have been found in any of the vast number of studies and clinical trials. Some cases people have taken 30 capsules a day with no ill effects.

Zyflamend

Another amazing supplement is Zyflamend, a combination of ten herbs for anti-inflammatory and anti-aging. I take it regularly to keep any inflammation away. Zyflamend has been the subject of ongoing research through Columbia University, the Cleveland Clinic and the M.D. Anderson Cancer Center.

Supplement Suggestions

- Serrapeptase – dosages vary for various conditions
- Digestive enzymes and bromelian
- Attokinase – helps to dissolve blood clots and lower blood pressure, origins: Japanese soybean
- ArthroMax – Life Extension formula contains glucosamine sulfate, theaflavins (black tea substance)
- Omega- 6 (gamma-linolenic acid)
- Multi-vitamin/mineral
- Anti-inflammatory herbs: boswellia (boswellia serrata), turmeric (curcuma longa), ginger (zingiber officinalis)
- Zyflamend

Immune Conditions

When the immune system is strong, we are protected from antigens (microorganisms, cancer cells, toxins). Antibodies (molecules) are produced to destroy antigens. Autoimmune disease occurs when the immune system is compromised. The body turns on itself and destroys normal body tissues. My mother's RA and Lupus were autoimmune diseases.

Vitamin C has long been considered an immune booster because it helps protect cells from free radical damage. Vitamin C intravenous therapy was introduced in the 1950's by Dr. Fredrick Klenner. Dr. John Meyers did further research on vitamin C IV's and the "Meyers' cocktail" was created.

A healthy immune system is influenced by our food choices, stress levels, lifestyles and airborne toxins. Carotenoids are a type of antioxidant found in green, red and yellow fruits and vegetables. In a double-blind study, after 15 days, those who received mixed carotenoids or beta carotene had significantly less DNA damage than those who did not. In an eight-week study, all groups who received carotenoid supplements showed less DNA damage.

Supplement Suggestions

• Vitamin C or "Meyers' cocktail"
• Glutathione
• Herbs: astragalus, echinacea, garlic, elderberry, cat's claw
• Vitamin E
• Zinc
• Probiotics
• Alpha- lipoic acid

Chemotherapy

Chemicals (antineoplastic) are used in an IV solution to help destroy cancer cells. Unfortunately besides killing abnormal cells, they also destroy normal cells. My sister had bladder cancer which metastasized into other organs and her brain. I would take her to chemo sessions. Afterwards, she would buzz with boundless energy until she crashed. Unfortunately the treatment made her more ill, and she died within six months. It was a painful process for her and very distressing for our family.

Supplement Suggestions

It is a known fact that all supplements, including vitamins and minerals, are discouraged while a person is on chemotherapy, as they are thought to counteract the effects of the therapy. Until more research can substantially support taking supplements while undergoing chemotherapy, it is advisable to consult with your oncologist.

Research

Unfortunately, new cancer drug research has been bogged down; it may take 10 to 20 years for pharmaceutical companies to seek and be awarded patents and FDA approvals. Our antiquated system has prevented more effective therapies from being approved while 1,500 Americans die each day from cancer.

Compassionate Access Act

There is a bill called The Compassionate Access Act of 2010 (H.R. 4732) which was introduced into Congress by The Abigail Alliance, a nonprofit organization. A 19-year-old girl, Abigail Burroughs, was diagnosed with squamous cell carcinoma of the neck and lungs. Her oncologist at John Hopkins Hospital wanted to use a new drug to help save her life. Unfortunately this drug hadn't been approved by the FDA even though it showed good responses in early trials. She was ineligible for the drug and after seven months of trying to get approval for its use, she passed away. Sadly, this drug was later approved for use against Abigail's form of cancer. The Compassionate Access Act would amend the Food, Drug and Cosmetic Act to approve drugs, biological products, and devices for seriously ill patients.

Complementary and Alternative Approaches

Complementary medicine works in complement with conventional medicine—radiation, chemotherapy and surgery. Alternative medicine uses other methods besides those mentioned. Clinical trial participation is available and eligibility requirements vary. Refer to the resource directory at the end of this book to obtain more information.

Complementary Therapies

- Herbal treatments – ginkgo, ginseng
- Acupuncture – alleviates nausea
- Massage – relief from pain, fatigue, depression and anxiety
- Yoga – helps strengthen and relax the body
-

- **Alternative Therapies**
- 714-X – a cocktail of chemicals that is said to stabilize your immune system so it can fight cancer
- Essiac – an herbal mixture with supposed antioxidant and anti-inflammatory effects. Refer to the author's book *Essiac: a Native Herbal Cancer Remedy*
- Gerson therapy – one of several treatments that are said to rid your body of cancer-causing toxins
- Liver flush – involves the drinking of juices and oils to cleanse the liver of cancer-causing agents
- Shark cartilage – used to hinder or stop the growth of cancer cells

Skin Cancer

There are three types of skin cancer: basal cell, squamous and melanoma, melanoma being the most serious form. Skin cancer is the most easily diagnosed and is primarily due to long unprotected exposure to the sun. Fair-skinned people are especially affected. Between 2 to 3 million people are diagnosed with non-melanoma cancer each year. Globally 132,000 melanoma cancers occur each year. According to Skin Cancer Foundation Statistics, one in five Americans will get skin cancer.

Cancer and the Sun

Two studies have shown that with the proper amount of vitamin D, risks of developing non-Hodgkin's lymphoma are reduced by 30 to 40%. This study included 3,000 lymphoma patients and 3,000 without lymphoma. Also, melanoma patients had less aggressive tumors and less likelihood of dying.

Remember to use common sense when sunbathing: avoid spending hours in the sun, use a natural sun screen, and stay out of the sun from 10:00 a.m. to 2:00 p.m. As mentioned earlier, Dr. Holick's studies have indicated that vitamin D is only produced during those hours so supplementing with vitamin D makes sense.

Supplement Suggestions

- Resveratrol
- Vitamin A
- Fernblock® supplement which helps shield skin from harmful ultraviolet rays
- Skin Eternal® by Source Naturals

High Blood Pressure (hypertension)

There are two measurements for registering blood pressure; systolic (pressure in arteries when heart beats) and diastolic (heart rests between beats). A normal reading is 120/80. Readings of 140/90 or higher is considered to be high blood pressure. If one has hypertension, heart disease is the number one cause of death. In the U.S. one to three adults have been diagnosed with hypertension. Many more may have high blood pressure but do not know it. Worldwide, one billion people have hypertension. That will rise to 1.56 billion by the year 2025. Factors that play a role in developing hypertension are heredity, aging, obesity, diet, tobacco and kidney failure (renal insufficiency). In the U.S., African–Americans are at a higher risk than Asians and Caucasians.

Supplement Suggestions

- Coenzyme Q-10
- Folic Acid – folate is a B vitamin which may help to lower high blood pressure in some people, possibly by reducing elevated homocysteine levels
- Fish oil – the DHA may help lower blood pressure
- Hawthorne
- Garlic – helps reduce systolic and diastolic levels if taking certain

blood thinners, gingko, and vitamin E

- Potassium
- Magnesium
- L-arginine
- Goldenrod
- Olive leaf
- Grapeseed

Low Testosterone

Male Hormones and Testosterone

Testosterone affects most organ systems; it is responsible for facial and body hair and muscle development. It also affects the nervous system, which is linked to aggression and risk-taking. Aging affects testosterone and estrogen levels in men. An enzyme called aromatase is involved in the production of estrogen. It acts by catalyzing the conversion of testosterone (an androgen) to estradiol (an estrogen). Aromatase is found in fat tissue; when men have excessive body fat, it can be an indicator that there is an excess of estrogen levels compared to testosterone.

Hormone Testing

After age 40 it is suggested that men be tested for both testosterone and estrogen along with having a complete physical exam. It is wise to have multiple testing done over time as hormone levels do vary widely among men. Saliva test kits provided by a certified laboratory will measure estradiol, progesterone, cortisol, testosterone, and DHEA.

Some side effects of a decrease in testosterone

- Depression
- Abdominal fat
- Lowered libido
- Heart disease
- Muscle mass decrease
- High blood pressure

- Diabetes
- Atherosclerosis
- Fatigue

Hormone Replacement for Men

There are precautions that should be taken with hormone replacement therapy as there may be contraindications such as the presence of prostate cancer. Certain hormone replacement therapies may contribute to the acceleration of such conditions. Work with a physician for prostate testing and careful monitoring of your hormone therapy.

Therapies to Increase Testosterone

There are many conventional and alternative therapies that a physician may prescribe to increase testosterone levels. They come in various forms; creams, patches, and sublingual tablets. The synthetic forms may produce side-effects which could include heart and kidney problems. Athletes have used this type of drugs for better performance and increased muscle mass. These therapies usually require a prescription. Natural therapies prescribed by alternative physicians include creams and sublingual tablets.

Suggested supplements

- Selenium – 200 mcg/day
- Vitamin A – 5000 IU/day
- Vitamin E – 400 IU/day plus 200 mg of gamma-tocopherol

Several supplements are recommended by Life Extension Foundation to complement hormone therapy.

- Acetyl-L Carnitine (1,000 to 2,000 mg/day)
- Chrysin (1,500 mg/day)
- Zinc (50 mg/day)
- Muira puama (850mg/day)
- Quercetin (500 to 1,000 mg/day)
- Saw palmetto (320 mg/day)

- Nettle root extract (240 mg/day)
- DHEA (15 to 75 mg/day with blood testing in 3-6 weeks)

It is strongly suggested that any supplements mentioned here should first be discussed with your physician regarding contraindications and suggested dosages.

Prostate Cancer and Hormones

Studies have revealed that higher levels of testosterone are not linked to prostate enlargement, whereas in older men estradiol (a form of estrogen) produces higher levels of estrogen in the prostate glands and can cause enlargement. Men who already show certain prostate conditions may show an increase in PSA (prostate-specific antigen) levels if on testosterone replacement therapy. If prostate disease has been diagnosed, testosterone therapy is contraindicated as it could cause an increase in cancer cells.

Life Extension Foundation recommends a program for men which you may wish to consider:

- Medical testing which includes blood levels PSA
- Testing free and total testosterone
- Aromatase inhibitors in the case of elevated estrogen levels
- Follow-up testing

The following suggestions may also be of benefit:

- Weight loss
- No alcohol (to help liver remove excess estrogen)
- Review all current medications being taken

In Closing

While growing up, sometimes I was asked to retrieve medicine for my parents and grandparents from their bathroom cabinets. I was always so amazed and mystified by the quantity of bottles which contained pills prescribed for various ailments. My mother was very careful not to give us prescriptions or over-the-counter remedies for colds, flu or other childhood ailments unless it was absolutely necessary. My brother, sister and I rarely became ill except for my sister's polio scare. My mother's cooking, spending summers at camp, being physically active and living in a relatively healthy environment all helped. In my junior year in high school I became sick. I had little energy, found it difficult to breathe and lacked focus to do most anything. For a couple of weeks I kept trying to convince my mother that something wasn't quite right with me. She always knew I was a healthy child so had difficulty believing me. Finally, at further insistence she took me to a general doctor who X-rayed my lungs and announced to my mother I had pleurisy, an infection in the lungs. He prescribed bed rest for 2 weeks. My mother felt so guilty that she hadn't listened to me that she transformed herself into "Florence Nightingale" during my recuperation period. I slept in her room during the day. She fed me bone marrow soup, broths, and the healthiest foods she could concoct. Naturally, I forgave her and was extremely grateful for her attentiveness.

As my own children had illnesses, I found myself answering a similar call of nursing. I always steered clear of pharmaceutical drugs and treated their childhood illnesses with herbs and various natural remedies. One time my son was taken to our Colorado small town general practitioner with an undiagnosed illness. It seemed serious. The doctor knew almost instantly that my son had encephalitis, a virus which can create acute inflammation of the brain. Trent was hospitalized and came home one week later fully recovered. I recognize that Western medicine can play a pivotal role, especially during a crisis situation.

This chapter has covered many health conditions and healthy suggestions. Use your wisdom in making choices when you have an illness and the true answers will come.

Half the modern drugs could well be thrown out the window, except that the birds might eat them.

–Martin H. Fischer

Deeper Than Skin Deep

When I was growing up, we played outside all day. There were no computers or television sets to keep us inside. Our mothers' warnings not to stay out in the sun fell on deaf ears. In college in the late 1950's, sunbathing became a ritual. We slathered on mixtures of baby oil and iodine and baked in the sun. Because of my Italian heritage my olive skin rarely burned, but my fair-skinned friends weren't so fortunate. We never used sunscreen (there was none). What were we thinking? I have read that taking good care of your skin should begin in your twenties—little did we know. As we grow older, perhaps we also grow wiser.

Skin and Your Health

We spend $43 billion annually on over 200 skin-care products and cosmetic procedures to make us look better, younger, and healthier. In 2005, North America spent $10 million on cosmetic surgery alone.

Our skin is the largest organ of our body. It weighs around 10 lbs. and covers an area of approximately 16 sq. feet. When we over-expose ourselves to sunlight, when we smoke or drink too much alcohol, when our eating habits are unhealthy, it is reflected in the condition of our skin. All these habits contribute to early aging of the skin: wrinkling, sagging, discoloration, and loss of elasticity. The condition of our skin also reflects our internal health.

Mirror, Mirror on the Wall

Have you looked at pictures of yourself when you were younger? I have, and I accept the fact that my hair is grayer, my skin less smooth and firm, and I see more lines. I have tried micro-dermabrasion, facials, and light peels. I have bought creams that guarantee to firm and plump up my sagging skin and lessen wrinkles and lines. Some products seem to bring better results than others, and some are terrifically expensive. I don't recommend the more expensive products because before we use them, we have no way of knowing how really effective they are or how much money we may be wasting.

Even with all the skin-care products and wrinkle-smoothing methods out there, good skin care boils down to this: exercise and nutritional programs, attitudes that we have about ourselves, and a choice of products that are free of chemicals and artificial ingredients. Are you positive? Are you stress-free? Do you laugh and fill yourself up with joy? Are you grateful for the good people and experiences in your life? Do you surround yourself with a loving family, partner and friends? Do you live each day to the fullest? Before bedtime I give thanks for five blessings I have received from my day. It has become a reminder of things I am grateful for. This practice is especially helpful when I have had a challenging day,

From the Inside Out

When we put clean, nutritious, organic (when possible) food into our bodies, our blood delivers healthy nutrients to all of our organs. Dark green leafy vegetables, raw or lightly steamed, help to flush out the toxins that build up in our liver, kidneys and intestines. When we watch our PH balance (by eating mostly alkaline foods) and exercise properly, the blood pumping through our system provides more strength and endurance, shorter recovery times and healthier blood cells.

Alcohol consumption, lack of exercise, drugs, acidic foods, and negative attitudes all contribute to harming and compromising our internal organs as well as our largest organ, our skin.

Dry Brushing & Moisturizing the Body

To help detoxify and invigorate your skin, start at your feet and brush towards your heart with a natural bristle brush. I enjoy dry brushing with a natural loofah-type brush before my shower and applying pure virgin coconut oil on my body, including my face and hair. Coconut oil is not only versatile in cooking, but applied topically it increases metabolism, heals injuries, and helps to smooth and firm the skin.

Pure virgin coconut oil is high in antioxidants that penetrate into the underlying tissues of our skin to prevent and protect against the formation of free radicals (which break down the skin's connective tissues as we age). The oil will also soften and moisturize skin while removing the outer layer of dead skin cells, making your skin smoother and more evenly textured with a healthy "shine." Be careful when purchasing body oils and lotions; many conventional body care products made with refined vegetable oils have all the antioxidants stripped from them (as a result of the refining process) and so are highly prone to free-radical generation, causing your skin to actually age faster.

Factors that promote early aging and wrinkling of the skin

- Smoking
- Skin type (people with light skin and blue eyes are more susceptible to sun damage)
- Heredity
- Occupational and recreational sun exposure over the course of many years
- Weight fluctuations
- Dehydration
- Lack of proper nutrients
- Poor diet
- Lack of exercise
- Stress
- Inadequate sleep
- Chemicals and drugs
- Toxins
- Hormone decline

Skin Care Basics

The main preventative measures to help us maintain a healthy body (both internally and externally) are; minimize excessive sun exposure; don't smoke; eat healthy foods; drink plenty of filtered water; reduce stress; and take anti-oxidants. We know that overexposure to the sun's UVB rays can damage the collagen and elastic fibers in the skin and create liver spots, wrinkles, rough and sagging skin—especially if we have spent years in the sun.

Sunscreens

The first true sunscreens came on the market in the early 1970's. The leading ingredient, PABA, was favored for binding readily to cells and for its water resistance. However, many people found it stained their clothing and some developed allergic reactions to this ingredient. It was later discovered that PABA may have been damaging to DNA. Obviously, few products today contain PABA, but we do have some smart choices of brands that are most beneficial and kinder to our older skin.

Safely Using Sunscreens

There has been some controversy about sunscreens. Are they safe to use and what kinds of sunscreens are better than others?

A majority of the sunscreens in the marketplace today contain one or more of the chemicals octyl methoxycinnamate (OMC), quarternium 15, DMDM hydantoin, and parabens. A study performed at the Norwegian Radiation Protection Authority in Oslo showed that the when the tissue culture of mice was exposed to a solution of OMC (far less than contained in sunscreens), it caused 50% of the cells to die, and when exposed to a sunlamp for two hours, more cells died, making the effect twice as toxic. When a sunscreen's purpose is to be used in the sun, what does that tell us about the safety of OMC?

Other chemicals besides OMC to look out for

• Benzophenone-3 (Bp-3)

• Homosalate (HMS)

• 4-methyl-benzylidene camphor (4-MBC)

• Octyl-dimethyl- PABA (OD-PABA)

• Octyl-methoxycinnamate

• Parabens (butyl-, ethyl-, methyl-, and propyl)

These chemicals are considered estrogenic; meaning any of several steroid hormones produced chiefly by the ovaries are responsible for promoting estrus and the development and maintenance of female secondary sex characteristics. They fool the body into believing they are naturally-produced hormones.

Two vital hormones that help to protect our skin are DHEA and melatonin. DHEA is an anti-stress hormone that helps safeguard against tissue destruction and accelerated aging by transporting essential nutrients through the blood stream. Topical use of DHEA performs 85 to 90% better than through supplementation. Melatonin is a sleep hormone and a free radical scavenger that enhances the skin's ability to repair free radical damage.

Sun Creams

I prefer going the chemical-free route in skin products; I find the more natural sunscreens much less irritating to my skin. I try not to put chemicals in my body, so why should I put them *on* my body, since the skin is the body's largest organ.

Here is a partial list of some sun products that are more beneficial and much kinder for your skin. Look for a natural sunscreen that protects from UVA (aging) and UVB (burning) rays with an SPF of at least 15 up to 30 SPF and use it year-around. These brands can often be found in your local health food store.

- Aubrey Organics® has an SPF 18 and 30 and Ultra Natural Herbal Sun Block
- Kiss My Face®, SPF 18 and 30
- Bronzo Sensuale®, SPF 30
- Lavera® (zinc oxide and titanium dioxide)
- Devita Daily Solar Protective Moisturizer ®(zinc oxide)
- Epicuren Discovery Zinc Oxide Sunscreen®
- JASON Naturals Sunbrellas Chemical-Free Sunblock ® (zinc oxide and titanium dioxide)
- All of these products are biodegradable. Most of these products contain similar ingredients: vitamins, antioxidants, shea butter, aloe vera, sesame oil, avocado oil, lanolin, zinc oxide, titanium dioxide (protects against UVA and UVB rays), and green tea (shown to protect against skin cancer)

In addition to putting sun creams on your skin, antioxidants will increase the body's ability to handle sun without burning. Astaxanthin is a powerful antioxidant that can be purchased at health food stores and is also found in shrimp, crawfish, lobster, and crab. It is an internal sunscreen that allows you to stay in the sun twice as long. Include vitamin C, green tea extract, or whole grape extract in your diet, and vitamin E lotion or pure vitamin E on your skin. Proper nutrition and plenty of pure water for hydration helps to keep the skin healthy.

Sun Tips

- Avoid burning
- Limit your sun exposure by staying out of the sun between 10:00 a.m. and 2:00 p.m.
- Allow sun exposure no more than two to three times weekly
- If you are not used to being in the sun, gradually build up your exposure beginning with 15 minutes a day and slowly increasing your time in the sun; fair-skinned people have a tendency to burn more easily because of the lower amount of melanin; I have been blessed with olive skin and tan easily
- Wear clothing that shields the sun's rays from the skin, or simply wear a long-sleeve shirt, long pants or skirt, hat and sunglasses
- People with dark pigmentation may actually tolerate 20 to 30 times more sun exposure than their fair-skinned counterparts

Skin Treatments

Skin treatments can be confusing; there are so many being touted as the best for eliminating wrinkles, firming the epidermis and boosting levels of collagen (a protein that works with elastin to give the body its tone and suppleness) that it's hard to sort it all out.

Treatments available for wrinkles include retinol (vitamin A), alpha hydroxy acids, antioxidants, lipid base serums and moisturizers. Medical cosmetic procedures include glycolic acid peels, deep peels, micro-derm-abrasion, laser resurfacing, surgical procedures (facelifts), Botox® injections, laser treatments and a multitude of new skin treatment choices which seem to appear daily. Of course, if you want to go all the way, cosmetic surgeons are always there. Take the time to find a reputable, board-certified cosmetic surgeon if surgery is in your future.

Facial Rejuvenation Acupuncture

While living in Hawaii I participated in a free session with several acupuncturists who were being taught how to apply needles on the face for rejuvenation. After the painless treatment, I decided to sign up for 12 weekly sessions with a locally trained acupuncturist to experience how my skin would improve in a healthier manner rather than submitting to cosmetic surgery procedures. Initially, the acupuncturist did a TCM (traditional Chinese medicine) diagnosis which is a done by checking the pulse, the tongue, and by observation. Not only were the sessions relaxing, but I also noticed my age spots lightening and my skin becoming rosier in color and feeling firmer.

Based on the principles of Oriental Medicine, acupuncture increases circulation throughout the blood and lymph system. Facial acupuncture helps the whole body look and feel younger by addressing the physical, mental and emotional patterns that cause disease and contribute to the aging process. Our skin ages for a number of reasons besides sun exposure: unhealthy diet, worry, overwork—all of which contribute to a depleted spleen, poor digestion and chronic infections. The health of our internal organs is also reflected in our outer appearance. For instance, if our kidneys are depleted, our bones and head are affected. Dark circles under our eyes may indicate a kidney imbalance. Dull skin indicates poor elimination.

While thousands of herbal formulations have been created throughout the 2,000-year history of acupuncture, few can equal the benefits of this ancient practice. Acupuncture is a very old science resulting in very youthful results.

There is an exact science with Chinese medicine. I would suggest studying up on this illuminating and fascinating subject.

The Treatment

Extremely fine needles are inserted into specific areas of the face. The entire procedure is relaxing and is usually done two times weekly in twenty to thirty minute sessions.

Benefits of Facial Acupuncture:

- Eliminates fine lines and diminishes wrinkles

- Improves muscle tone and dermal contraction and tightens pores
- Increases collagen production
- Eliminates and reduces bags under the eyes and lifts drooping eyelids
- Decreases sagging
- Reduces or eliminates double chins
- Eliminates puffiness
- Improves skin color
- Brightens the eyes
- Reduces stress evident in the face
- Enhances innate beauty and radiance

Precautions

If you are pregnant or experiencing allergic reactions, have herpes, a cold or the flu, wait until the symptoms subside and consult with the practitioner before initiating sessions. This treatment may not be for you if severe conditions exist such as high blood pressure or diabetes, or if you are using anticoagulants including aspirin or coumadin®. If you have had recent laser resurfacing or micro-dermabrasion, allow one to three months before facial acupuncture treatments.

Skin Care for Mature Skin

As we age, our skin becomes increasingly rough and wrinkled and may show some irregular pigmentation (coloration). All this is due to the natural decrease in our body's production of collagen and elastin. Our skin requires different care with age. As we grow older, our skin doesn't produce new cells at the same pace. Environmental and biological factors take their toll. We often develop enlarged pores, and the effects of the sun become evident in age spots, wrinkles and freckles. Our desire is to replenish dry, sensitive and aging skin in the most beneficial method made available.

There are a staggering 1,000-plus chemicals and preservatives that you want to avoid, and many of them are present in mainstream over-the-counter cosmetic and skin care products. In 2003 the European Commission banned most of these chemicals from beauty products. In the U.S., the Food and Drug Administration (FDA) has lagged behind, only banning nine of the hundreds of chemicals from cosmetic products. There is, however, a website you can access for information on companies who have signed a pledge not to use the European-banned chemicals. Remember, our skin is the largest organ in the body and absorbs everything we put on it; it seems to make sense to use the freshest and most pure ingredients possible, doesn't it?

Some pure lines I like

MyChelle Dermaceuticals® based in Frisco, Colorado
Juice Beauty® certified organics
Emerita® skincare products
Jurlique® products

All these lines contain 100% certified organic vegetable ingredients free of parabens, synthetic fragrances and petroleum derivatives. The Juice concentrates contain antioxidants, vitamins and essential nutrients. None of these companies charge exorbitant prices.

Exfoliating

Exfoliating skin daily helps cellular turnover, stimulates collagen and removes dry skin which prepares the skin for a water-base serum and moisturizing cream with an SPF 30. Avoid petroleum and lanolin ingredients as they clog the skin. I discovered a 10% glycolic cream at the health store which I apply once daily, usually at night. I also use a vitamin C serum with 28% concentrate each morning before applying my moisturizer and sunscreen. Twice monthly, I apply a 50% lactic acid peel. It is wise to start with a lower percentage and gradually build up until your skin becomes adjusted. This helps with cellular turn over and exposes newer, fresher, more youthful skin. I wash with a Clarisonic® brush which cleans the face using a micro-massage action. According to clinical studies, when used properly it removes makeup six times better than manual facial cleansing, cleans pores and makes skin products more absorbable and effective.

There are a myriad of wonderful skin creams available. Explore, research and discover how you can have healthier and more radiant youthful looking skin without paying a premium price. Find out which ones work for your particular skin type. I suggest you find a local esthetician that you trust to help you decide which treatments and products are best for you.

If you are fortunate enough to live in a moist climate rather than a dryer high-altitude or desert climate, your skin can feel like velvet. If you do live in a dry climate, use a humidifier, and frequently mist and moisturize your skin. Remember to drink plenty of filtered water, limit sun exposure between the hours of 10:00 a.m. and 2:00 p.m., use a safe sunscreen every day, and most of all be happy and enjoy your life!

Spas: More Than Skin Deep

A weekend at a spa could easily cost $500 or more for lodging, meals, a few treatments and perhaps a class or two. Spa-goers want more than just the massage experience. We want advice on how to maintain and improve our skin through products, nutrition and techniques that we can use in our own home.

The Perfect Spa in Your Own Home

There are resources at the back of the book to help you select a good spa in your area.

You can treat yourself to a spa day in the comfort of your own home. Begin your day with silence and a stretch. Soak in a lavender-scented bath—a great stress reliever. Adding sea salts also helps to detoxify the body. Light candles and turn off the phone. Give yourself a facial by blending oatmeal and milk in a blender to make a paste and apply it to your clean face. This mask helps to draw out toxins and increase circulation. Soak two steeped chamomile tea bags in ice-cold milk and place on eyelids for 10 minutes to reduce puffiness and rejuvenate tired eyes. Eat light and healthy foods. Take a walk. Read a book or watch a funny movie.

The information in this section is intended to act only as a guide. Each of us has our own skin type, our own lifestyles and attitudes. Do not try to compare yourself to friends, strangers or models in magazines. Do not be too easily influenced by "miracle" anti-aging medical procedures. Create your own identity and be a most beautiful, compassionate friend to yourself.

— Step 6 —

Take Charge of Your Finances: Health & Home

How I Developed Passion for a Healthy Life Style

As you know, I watched my mother suffer from rheumatoid arthritis (an autoimmune disease) while I was growing up and saw that none of the prescriptions she was given for her pain and swelling 50 years ago helped to improve her debilitating disease. While I was in college, I received a phone call from my mother. She had fallen while getting out of her tub, had snapped her hip, and was in the hospital awaiting surgery. She was 45 at the time. She tried to explain to me what had happened; however, the medications and the fall were causing hallucinations—she said there were creatures under her hospital bed and she was frightened and couldn't understand why she was in the hospital. After trying to soothe her, I called my family and demanded to know why I wasn't told my mother was in the hospital. The response was "we didn't want to worry you." This was the standard line for various family situations that arose.

After hip surgery, my mother refused physical therapy and never walked again. She later contracted lupus, had a stroke and passed away at 52 years of age. My father, who was 9 years older, had been her caregiver. As a family we were never informed of his own blood disorder. My father was a very private man and never discussed his health with his children. My parents passed away within six weeks of one another. I felt a profound sense of loss—especially because they had died so young. There were never any preventative or alternative treatments considered for my parents during that time. The prescribed drugs may have eased my mother's severe pain and joint swelling, but the side effects created severe depression and I believe eventually led to the onset of lupus and premature death.

Thus, in my mid-twenties, after my parents' passing, I began my quest for alternative healing. All these years later I continue along my path of well-being through Chinese doctors, regular massages, and contacting a naturopathic doctor in my area if certain health conditions arise. I do not take prescription drugs unless it is absolutely necessary. I prefer complementary medicine and have for many years. I have changed my nutritional habits throughout the years, continue to exercise and pursue core strengthening activities such as yoga, Pilates and dance. I manage the stress of everyday living through breath work, meditation, and gratitude for the blessings I receive each day. Today's medicine and healing has come a long way since my parents' time.

The New Medicine

PBS aired a documentary in March of 2006 entitled *The New Medicine*. The show was hosted by Dana Reeve, who was later diagnosed with lung cancer following the death of her actor husband, Christopher Reeve. Sadly, Dana passed away shortly after her husband's death, although reports stated she was not a cigarette smoker.

The show focused on mainstream, traditional doctors and medical departments not known for being "cutting edge" or "alternative/complementary." The cameras went into healthcare clinics, private practices and research institutions to illustrate a new movement taking place in medical clinics and hospitals around the country; to treat the patient as a whole person and consider, among other things, their lifestyle, culture, and stress factors.

The medical community is beginning to recognize the importance of their patients' desires to get well and place more emphasis on prevention rather than treating a patient with a disease-based protocol. Many hospitals are integrating complementary modalities like acupuncture into their systems. The Latin root word for doctor means teacher. A pro-active physician can help a patient avoid disease by teaching them how to take better care of themselves through preventative measures. This progressive outlook presents a new medical paradigm in health care and prevention of disease. Since 1948, the United Nations World Health Organization definition of health has been "an active state of complete physical, mental and social well-being."

A new era in preventative medicine has emerged. Founded in 1995, the World Academy of Anti-Aging and Regencrative Medicine (WAAM) makes available to physicians (M.D.s) and Osteopaths (D.O.s) fellowships, extensive course training, and studies in age management and regenerative medicine. This knowledge is also available to institutions, researchers and accredited universities throughout the world. Understanding how cells function and regenerate tissues and organs can represent a revolutionary breakthrough for people around the globe. Age Management consists of individualized evaluations and testing which include hormone levels, nutrition, brain cognitive testing and physical performance. Through physical exams and performance testing, these customized programs can assist in improving one or more of the following conditions or symptoms; excess weight, lack of muscle tone, low libido, hormonal imbalances, and impaired cognitive processes..

Regenerative Medicine

Wake Forest University Baptist Institute for Regenerative Medicine, created in 2004, offers new medical research and leading-edge bioengineering. This is the largest facility in the world in its field; it has more than 150 scientists devoting their expertise toward developing organs for transplant into the bodies of people. These organs range from bladders to heart valves and arteries. The blood and the cells of the patients are placed into a mold of the organ or body part and incubated. Anthony Atala, M.D., the Director of the institute, has had long-term success and improvement in the lives of children and teenagers who have received new bladders from these advanced procedures. My sister was diagnosed with bladder cancer and at the time, the doctor's answer was to remove her bladder. She refused because she was adamant not to carry around an ostomy bag for the remainder of her life.

Hyperbaric Chamber

I read that the performer Michael Jackson had his own hyperbaric chamber. If we could all afford to have one, we may be healthier for it. The pressure in a hyperbaric chamber causes the oxygen to dissolve into all of the body fluids so that the red blood cells and blood plasma becomes drenched with oxygen. Plasma carries extra oxygen to areas where circulation is poor or blocked, by trickling past the blockages or by seeping into the areas that the red blood cells are too large to reach. Plasma is made up of smaller particles than red blood cells. This extra oxygen provides the extra energy needed in the healing process. New capillaries are formed which aid in healing wounds, autism, brain function, cerebral palsy, poor circulation and gangrene to name some of the physical benefits.

Dr Edgar End was most prominent and knowledgeable on hyperbaric benefits as a clinical professor of Environmental Medicine at the University of Wisconsin Medical School; he noted:

"I've seen partially paralyzed people half carried into the (HBOT) chamber, and they walk out after the first treatment. If we got to these people quickly, we could prevent a great deal of damage."

A person lies in the pressurized glassed chamber which provides a 360 degree view. The treatment lasts up to an hour, and there may be music or even television provided. There are solo hyperbaric chambers, chambers that hold two people, and group chambers. If you are interested, you can do a little research in your area to see what is available.

Infrared Saunas

While living in Hawaii, I was most fortunate to often be able to use an infrared sauna. It was situated on some property owned by a woman who had a small natural healing center. The sauna was located outside. The unit contained several fiberglass carbon infrared heaters, a bench, and windows. I would sit inside for 20 to 30 minutes allowing the heat to absorb into my body. I was able to control the temperature from inside. Research indicates heat can absorb more than 1.5" into the body. Sitting in the sauna can help reduce toxins and help burn calories equivalent to running 2 to 3 miles. After my session I would walk a few feet to a lovely Hawaiian outdoor shower area to rinse off, feeling refreshed and energized.

The Healing Machine

While wandering the downtown streets of San Clemente, California, I spotted a sign that read "Health Center." In the store I was introduced to a space-age looking machine called Turbosonic®. It was developed, patented and introduced in Germany. After decades of research and development, the machines are now in the U.S. with FDA approval. A person stands on a platform while receiving sonic vibrations at different frequencies. Various levels of vibration can be set to improve medical conditions such as emphysema, osteoporosis, arthritis and rheumatism, multiple sclerosis and lower back pain. Results are felt in as little as 10 minutes on the machine. It replaces an hour and half of conventional exercise for muscle development, core conditioning and weight loss. It increases cellular oxygen circulation while moving cellular waste out of the body. Other benefits include improved balance, coordination, and flexibility. I experienced lower back pain on my road trip from Colorado to California. In one session my back pain disappeared, I felt more energized during the day, and slept soundly at night. To access in-depth studies, refer to the resources at the back of this book.

Taking Steps Toward Improved Health

How can you actively participate in addressing your health concerns as well as implement preventative steps for a long and healthy life? You can contact WAAM or locate a practitioner in your area who may be recommended by a friend or another wellness professional. Continue to educate yourself about alternative and complementary procedures through the excellent magazines, books and web resources available. Massage, acupuncture, herbs, and infrared saunas are only a few of the modalities available today that help to complement your whole picture of health and vitality. Find a health practitioner whom you trust. Locate physicians who are educating themselves in different healing modalities to supplement traditional medical care and the customary reliance on prescription pharmaceuticals. Acupuncture and massage therapy helps treat such conditions as back pain or stress-related illnesses and can be far less expensive through an alternative practitioner.

Steps to Your Financial Future

I grew up in a conservative East Coast family. My father was an engineer who received a free college scholarship at Cooper Union College in New York City. My mother had a business degree, and my grandfather was a college graduate from Italy. My grandmother quit school after eighth grade and worked to support her Italian mother who did not speak English. She lived with my grandparents helping to raise her two daughters, my mother and aunt. My grandfather's first wife had died after giving birth to my aunt. She was not able to read or write well nor did she ever drive a car. Her husband, on the other hand, was a graduate of New York University. His father had died at an early age leaving his wife to raise a number of children, many of whom were able to work their way through college.

My Italian grandparents were an enterprising couple who developed a plastics company in 1918 in the U.S., and their hard work over next 35 years provided them a comfortable life. We could have lived in large elegant homes, driven expensive cars, worn expensive clothes and jewelry and traveled around the world, but my family did not believe in spending money on possessions. As young adults my brother, sister and I didn't expect to live in the lap of luxury. We were happy. My parents' idea of redecorating wasn't buying new furniture and "things" for our home but to put the winter drapes away and hang the lighter summer ones and put summer slipcovers on the living room furniture. Because my father was an engineer he was a master at fixing broken things. (He remodeled a section of the basement as our play area.)

Our Christmas gifts were ice skates, sleds, mittens, clothes, a new bike and a few toys. We had two cars for my parents but I rode my bicycle to school every day. We saved money for necessities like doctor and dental checkups, school, food and clothing. We had a freezer which held meats and poultry. Food didn't spoil and get thrown away. We didn't have a dishwasher so after each evening meal my sister and I would wash and dry dishes. My brother sometimes managed to sneak off before putting them away. My sister and I shared a bedroom which was a converted attic. We held down summer jobs during high school, were fortunate to be given college educations, and were taught values and principles. My parents and grandparents always lived within their means. They only bought homes without mortgages and while some of our friends' parents were spending beyond their resources and in debt, we lived without any fear of collapse. My grandparents donated money to colleges, hospitals and an orphanage in the Italian town where my grandfather grew up. My grandfather didn't invest in the stock market, but chose instead to develop and invest in real estate which brought him great rewards. It was a period in life when people were enterprising, worked hard and were practical. Families were of primary importance. To this day I detest excess or waste in my life.

My Career Challenges

Carolyn Myss is an international author and speaker who has an interesting take on job descriptions during our lifetimes. In our earlier years Carolyn's belief is that our work is called a 'job'. Perhaps as a college graduate we are testing the deeper waters outside the classroom. My first job after college was as an elementary school teacher. I was following my major as an educator but it fell short of my expectations in a short time. Following that brief experience, I took a hum-drum job in a credit bureau office in Washington DC where my organization and people skills were finely honed. I was paid more than the other girls just because I had a college diploma.

During the 1950's and 1960's many women were expected to attend college, get married, have children and become homemakers similar to Julie Robert's depiction of a 1950's college teacher in the movie *Mona Lisa Smile*. While in my twenties, my husband and family moved to Snowmass, Colorado. I purchased my first affordable retail business which was a small kitchen shop in the middle of a mountain village. Shortly after that, my sister-in-law became my business partner. During the next four years, I learned about buying items, displaying, and managing finances. Then suddenly, a messy and traumatic divorce forced me to sell my business and move. Today, looking back on that pivotal time in my life, being a single mother of three young children, I remember feeling rocked to the core and that I had very little worth or self-esteem. I was in my early 30s and inexperienced in coping with this major episode I never anticipated.

My decision to remarry a year later was built on my still rocky foundation and feelings of desertion stemming from my previous marriage. My second husband had custody of his two young boys. My world was tilting left and right with five small children ranging in age from four to ten to take care of. During the next eight years I held part-time jobs to help provide a more even keel and balance between the multitude of motherly duties in a full house, finding me amongst all of the activity, and making the marriage work. Alcoholism tore the relationship apart, and once again I took the next steps into the void.

However, this time was different. My children were older; I was braver and more self assured. I was also grateful that my parents weren't still living to witness their middle daughter's dramas. After all, my two siblings and I felt we were raised to maintain certain standards in life, being the best in all ways possible. A year went by while my husband vacillated about signing the divorce papers; I lived in a townhome with my youngest daughter who was graduating from high school, and took a job with a small company which erected parking garages. Nine months later, and coping with daily migraines, I was told that the company was cutting back on expenses, and because I was the new employee they had to let me go.

This was a true blessing and turning point in my life. My youngest daughter graduated from high school, I moved to California with a new business partner and then, into my 40s, I launched the second phase of my work experience. I began to sense a higher purpose. Carolyn Myss calls this the 'career' stage of our lives. The career of importing natural health products for an Australian company catapulted me into new realms of experience and self confidence. My interest and research in natural health for many years helped to prepare me for this new venture. My children were grown and no longer living at home, which afforded me time to fully concentrate on my business. The next four years were an exciting and fulfilling time. The business prospered but came to a screeching halt when the Australian company decided to move their offices to the states and offer us a smaller position which we sensed would not last. We felt devastated. For several months the attorneys bickered, and walked away with more money in their pockets than we did. Starting over again was an agonizing thought—how and where? Neither my partner nor I had saved much money as it was put back into our business venture.

A year later, through innumerable tears, anguish and prayers, another opportunity opened for me, and at age 46 I found myself stepping through the doorway which Carolyn Myss calls your third stage; your 'vocation'. I decided to begin writing a book on Australian tea tree oil, an Australian herb. In 1990, my new book publishing venture began and through the period of the next 12 years I wrote and published more books and helped a few other authors do the same. Much of my direction came from reading voluminous amounts of publishing material, attending workshops and using my sixth sense. I felt for the first time a real sense of purpose, enthusiasm and fulfillment. There were a few unfortunate experiences along my path, however. One of my authors absconded with 20 cases of books out of my office while I was away on Christmas holiday. She had been under contract granting her the rights to buy her books for her own marketing. She never responded to any of my calls for payment. Hiring an attorney was economically unfeasible for me at the time. I contacted a publishing remaining company in New York City (a remaining company purchases books from publishing houses at a deep discount and sells them at a cost below the original retail). We agreed upon a price they would pay my company and the rest of the stock of the books were shipped east.

Another difficult lesson came from a children's book project. This project contained stories and beautiful photographs of impoverished children around the world. It was a giant step from my traditional genre of natural healing but I became enthralled with the idea and the financial opportunities it could afford me. The book would be presented on national television with the possibility of the celebrated Oprah Winfrey producing and narrating a television special. Of course my head was swirling with endless possibilities. The author and I agreed to a contract and she whisked off to Europe for a book symposium with marketing material in hand, which my business provided.

The floor collapsed upon her return. She informed me that she was going to cancel the contract and take it to another publishing house. She even told the woman photographer whose images she was using for the book that she found another photographer. As it happened, she met a male photographer at the conference, fell madly in love with him, and was going to have him take over the photographic project. The entire episode lasted for a few months, causing me much humiliation and distress but I had to move on. In retrospect I realized I had allowed my ambition and success to get in the way of sound reasoning.

Ponzi Scheme

During the time in which my business was going through the challenges I mentioned, a friend approached me about an investment group that was paying back dividends up to 20%. She had received a great amount off of her original investment. I was unaware of Ponzi schemes at the time, and I trusted her. Here again, greed and perhaps desperation played a part in my decision to invest some savings into the investment group. I do recall when writing the check that things did not feel right, but I mailed the money anyway. Shortly after that, the Ponzi scheme came to a screeching halt. I never received a dime back. I discovered afterwards that people like my friend were being paid dividends off of the latest investors' money and when the time was ripe the schemers shut the business down, hid the money leaving the investors at a total monetary loss. A class action suit was brought but because there were many people in the investment group throughout the U.S., very little money was recovered to be dispersed among the group. I spoke to an artist from Manhattan who had lost over $200,000. One of the men behind the Ponzi scheme was a medical doctor who was wheelchair bound. He was indicted along with some other people. Although these experiences were painful at the time, I learned a great deal more about myself during those trying times. Resiliency and optimism played a positive part in my emotional recovery. And I found I was able to forgive myself and others in order for me to continue down the path.

The vocation stage in my life has represented the culmination of years of work achievements and experiences which now give rise to a higher purpose. For instance, I had been drawn to natural health for over 30 years. That interest propelled me through various jobs as a health food manager, product importer, researcher, health writer, author and publisher. I believe we all have unique callings during our lifetime. I have immense gratitude for teachers and even the heartache experiences that have crossed my path throughout these years. What is your calling?

"The whole purpose of education is first to prepare you with essential knowledge for the next stage in your life and then to persuade,

coerce and convince you to use that knowledge in the hope that you
will not, because of ignorance, be a destructive force to yourself and
to others. Of course you will forget details and facts, but all these
years of learning in the areas of human knowledge will compel you
nevertheless to remember at least where essential knowledge is to be
found, or even re-discovered when you need it"

~ *PEARL BUCK*

Grown Children: Their Family and Finances

My grown children struggle more than I did during my formative years. They are faced with a climate of challenging economic times while they raise their children, have jobs and find valued time to spend with themselves and their husbands. They have told each other that they didn't learn about finances from their parents while growing up; they had to learn this for themselves. From my perspective, we had them work during the summers, have an allowance, and tried to be sensible toward how money was spent. Looking back, I think more could have been done to demonstrate and teach them about finances and managing money. My husbands were both spendthrifts which didn't help matters either. I found myself taking over the role of budgeting and paying the monthly bills. Finances and raising a family still was a challenge on many levels.

My eldest granddaughter recently graduated from a Colorado college. She told me that she has learned the value of money by having jobs throughout her four-year education. Her father has employed her and his son during school holidays and summer in his business. This is positive training for the working world which awaits them. Changes and challenges are to be expected in our lifetime. How we choose to deal with new opportunities and move forward is testament to our true self. Can we live each day with positive and realistic attitudes or dive into a cavernous hole of despair and fear?

Barn's burnt down ~ now I can see the moon

~ *MASAHIDE (1657-1732), TRANSLATED BY LUCIEN STRYK*

The Nature of Today's Financial World

In today's world we find ourselves clinging to a precarious precipice. As

I was writing this book in early spring 2009, the U.S. had experienced the greatest economic crisis in the financial industry since the Great Depression. Americans cast their deciding votes for the young African American Illinois Senator who was elected the 44th President of the United States.

Barack Obama inherited a massive and volatile economic recession which had been accelerating in 2007. In 2010, 1.52 million people declared bankruptcy. Several major mortgage companies went bankrupt, and unemployment became the highest in 40 years. The war in Iraq and Afghanistan were still raging on, food and gasoline prices soared, home foreclosures were occurring at an alarming rate and the banking and financial industries suffered catastrophic losses—many went bankrupt. The World Bank reported that 129 countries were experiencing a shortfall of $270 billion to $700 billion in 2009, making the world economic picture greatly challenged and in crisis.

These have become very difficult times for people worldwide who are losing their jobs and desperately trying to hold onto their homes and retirement investments. The U.S. unemployment rate rose to 10% in 2010. In June, 2011, the rate was 9.5% with 15 million still unemployed. The International Labour Organization has reported that there could be a loss of 51 million jobs worldwide. The International Monetary Fund warns that poverty and violence is on the increase in third world countries. The world feels like it is teetering on its edge attempting to be brought upright in more loving balance.

The Baby Boomer Generation Grows Up

While Boomers may want to be young, they know they are getting older and need to plan accordingly. However, only 15% of Boomers believe they are saving enough money to cover their future needs. Many Boomers do not look forward to a leisurely retirement. The 2005 data revealed that saving for retirement was an important but not overwhelming factor for most Boomers. The key goals included saving for unexpected emergencies and future medical problems, as well as saving for major purchases and fun activities, such as vacations. Our society tends to be very good at procrastination, and as a result, many Boomers will find themselves, by necessity, working at a post-retirement age. The life expectancy of a healthy adult at age 65 is 80 years. There is a good chance that one of the spouses in a marriage will live beyond that, perhaps to 90 or more. The greatest risk is that they'll outlive their money.

The rule of thumb is to project post-retirement income at 75% of pre-retirement income. For example, if a couple earns $100,000 pre-retirement, $75,000 should meet their needs in retirement. The question is then "what level of assets would support a $75,000 income?"

Based on a Monte Carlo Simulation (a technique that uses random numbers and probability to solve problems), the amount of available assets should be approximately $1.5 million to $2 million in order to provide an income of $75,000 per year. Let me explain further.

The Monte Carlo Simulation gives a framework that tells us how long your money will last given the rate of return on the money compared to the amount and rate of withdrawal. In simple terms, if you withdraw a higher percent than you are earning, at some point you will run out of money. Over the last 100 years the Standard and Poor's Index has averaged about a 10% return on investment. The index is comprised of 100% of large-capitalization stocks which represent the largest portion of the economy; i.e., IBM®, Coca-Cola®, Microsoft®, Proctor and Gamble®, etc.

The average retiree should not hold all assets in stocks, but should have a balanced combination of stocks, fixed income investments (bonds, CDs, etc.), and a certain percentage in cash in a savings account or money market fund. Typically, an average retiree should have the following asset allocation: 50 to 60% in stocks, 30 to 35% in fixed income and the balance in savings.

As a result of this allocation, projected future returns could potentially be in the range of 7 to 8%. Going back to the assets available to generate these returns, as a rule of thumb, you could withdraw 4 to 5% of the return. The balance of the return should be reinvested in order to grow the assets to keep pace with inflation.

Simply put, if your portfolio is earning a total return of 8% and you are withdrawing 5%, there is a 3% surplus which is reinvested back into your portfolio, allowing the assets to grow. Remember, one of the spouses may live far beyond the average life expectancy, and as a result you not only need to preserve your assets, but grow them.

The information in the section on Baby Boomer economics was contributed by my brother, Robert Baldanza. Robert was a financial advisor with a major brokerage firm and had been in the financial services business since 1970. He is now retired and lives in Florida with his wife of 43 years.

Inheritance

According to a recent study of the Federal Reserve Board's Survey of Consumer Finances by the American Association of Retired People, about 85% of Boomers expect to inherit nothing. 92% of the general population will receive no inheritance; 4% will receive $25,000 or less; and only 1% of the population can expect to receive over $100,000 with the remaining 2/5 receiving between $25,000 and $100,000. It's becoming increasingly obvious that we cannot rely on family money, and the worldwide economic picture has put a stress on retirement accounts, company pensions and investments to secure our future.

About ten years ago I took a finance course from a woman whose father had a well known U.S. company that helped people prepare and file their yearly taxes. Her father was a professional icon in his field and yet when she had questions surrounding money she was told not to be concerned. As a result, she didn't comprehend how to manage her own assets until two husbands spent much of her wealth. It was at this point in her life she made the decision to learn everything she could about finances, wrote a book about her experience, and began to lecture and hold seminars for women around the country. We can continue to educate ourselves on how to manage and be smart with our money. There are many resources available on the internet, books and financial courses.

Simplify

One way to manage our money is to simplify our life. A local Denver news show told of an elderly woman who had lived on her property near train tracks and enjoyed the sounds of the trains going by only to have her home destroyed by a fire which was caused by sparks from a passing train. A couple of years before, she had turned down an offer of $1 million from a real estate developer. She said that she had no desire to sell. This was her home and she planned on staying there for the remainder of her life. All her possessions had been lost in the fire. What drew my attention was when asked by a reporter how she was coping in losing everything she responded "You never see a person in Heaven with a U-Haul."

How can we choose to be more at peace in today's complex and anxious world? I made the decision to scale down financially and incorporate living more simply. While the cost of living has risen I have had to learn to become a more conscious consumer.

Keys to Simplify

- Charge on a credit card only what can be paid off each month
- Budget monthly money carefully
- Buy clothes and household items at thrift and second hand stores
- Sell personal items on EBay® and Craig's List®.
- Consign expensive jewelry and antiques to help put more money into savings
- Clean out closets every few months and either consign the contents or donate to a local thrift store
- Household items not saleable can go to organizations like Habitat for Humanity®
- Shop for food more often, buying smaller quantities of produce that will be used in a few days
- Look for items on the grocery shelf that are discounted
- During the summer months, frequent local farmers markets
- Recycle and conserve on energy by biking rather than driving your car everywhere
- Use more blankets on your bed during the colder months while lowering the thermostat
- During the summer months plant a garden to provide some fresh vegetables, herbs and fruit
- In the warmer months have your family and friends enjoy the splendor of a summer evening with a picnic while listening to free music concerts

Do not make despair your focus; rather have hope, gratitude and love for the blessings you receive each day. Use these times to change things in your life that no longer serve. Simplify, reach out to family and friends and know that a positive attitude will bring you a brighter tomorrow.

Consider Relocating

I have lived from the east coast of the U.S. to the Hawaiian Islands. Some of the moves were related to job opportunities while others I found geographically appealing. My parents, grandparents, aunts, uncles and siblings didn't move around. I was the adventurer and the nomad. I have kidded my brother and his family that if they ever decide to move out of the home they have lived in for over 30 years, it may take them another 30 to sort through all of their worldly possessions. When we move around we don't have the time or ability to accumulate a lot of stuff. Living in various places has made me appreciate meeting new people and making friends along the way. The scenery changes and it opens up new doors for me to walk through.

I have hiked the Olympic Peninsula in the Northwest, seen eagles nest, taken ferries to Canada and kayaked along the shores. In Hawaii I swam in the warm Pacific waters, kayaked alongside the dolphins and watched the whales breach. I have shopped at outside farmers markets, picked tropical flowers for my home and listened to the beautiful Hawaiian music. In Colorado, I ski with my family, plant my vegetable garden, have lawn picnics at summer music concerts, watch the first snowfall of the winter, sit by a beautiful river and bike and hike the trails. Perhaps none of these experiences would have happened for me if I had chosen to live in one place. Moving around is not for everyone, but for me it has been enchanting, exhilarating and liberating. The idea of relocating is a lifestyle choice for many. The factors may be based on economics, health or simply the desire to live elsewhere.

Population Growth and Demographics

As I was completing this section of the book, news agencies announced that the U.S. population was officially at over 300 million people. The U.S. population hit 200 million in 1967 and has grown 50% since that time, while production of goods and services accelerated by 217%. In 35 years, our population is projected to be 400 million, including (legal) immigrants. Baby Boomers will be replaced with younger taxpayers, and the increased population will hopefully keep our economy thriving.

Even with the projected increase, the U.S. will still have only one-sixth the population density of Germany, for instance, whose population is expected to stop growing within a few years. Some U.S. states are also experiencing a decrease in population. Currently North Dakota, Ohio, Kansas and Nebraska average fewer than 14 households per square mile. A decrease in population will have an effect on the economy of those states and nations, as they must depend on younger generations to fill the economic gap.

According to The Center for Environment and Population, a nonpartisan research group in New Canaan, Connecticut, more than half the population of this country currently lives within 50 miles of the coasts. In a decade, with an additional 25 million people, half the total population increase will also be residing near the coasts. Along with this projected increase in population over the next decade, there will be an emergence of mega-cities, and 25 million more people will be seeking employment.

What impact this density will have on the environment is yet to be seen. Fragile water supplies in the desert areas of the Southwest may be affected, and low-lying areas of the southern states may be prone to hurricanes and massive flooding such as that experienced with Hurricane Katrina in 2005. States such as Colorado, Montana and Northern California may experience diminished water supplies in their rivers. Personally, I have witnessed a population explosion in the last 20 years along the Colorado Western slope especially in the resort towns where more affluent people are seeking land and mountain properties.

We are also experiencing an increase in the number of Hispanics throughout the country. Expensive housing and costly real estate may drive less affluent people inland in the future. Tennessee's Hispanic population, for instance, is up 140%. By mid-century, when my grandchildren are between the ages of 44 and 62, the 34% population increase in the United States will have affected demographics, the environment, jobs, water supplies, energy distribution, and every other aspect of life, including retirement options.

Various regions within America indicate various personalities according to an extensive study done by Cambridge University. Extroverts are found more often in the Southeast, Midwest and Great Plain states. Creative and open minded people are living in the Northeast and on the West Coast. More neurotic people may reside from Maine to Louisiana. Conscientious people tend to live in the South or Midwest. People may have a tendency to move to areas where they feel more comfortable; where they will fit in. Some may value the newness of an area in which they can reshape their thinking and develop new ideas of living and incorporate that into their health, occupations and academic world.

Where Do You Want to Live?

Based on a survey of 450,000 adults, Colorado, New Mexico and Hawaii capture 3 of the 10 top spots where 59-plus Americans can expect to live longest. How fortunate for me that I live in Colorado, and am able to be in Hawaii during the winter months. There are currently over 500 centenarians in Colorado who have several surprising things in common regarding their lifestyles. They enjoy exercise and lots of sunshine (which all three of these states get plenty of); their diets are low in carbohydrates (which means more protein); they enjoy 2 to 3 ounces of alcohol intake per day, take multi-vitamins, and most have better-than-average educations (they're smart). There are small cities and towns that are rated each year in AARP Bulletin Magazine. You can access all that information by going to their website. Check the Resource section at end of this book.

Elder hostels

In 1975, Marty Knowlton was the co-founder of this international educational organization. He passed away in 2009 at age 88, leaving behind an incredible legacy. Elder hostels can be found in the 50 U.S. states and over 90 countries. The not-for-profit provides over 8,000 educational programs in which over 160,000 people 55 years and older have participated. Ideas are exchanged through lectures, field trips and travels. Many participate in hiking, photography, opera, birding and water sports.

Living Outside of the U.S.: Retirement Advantages

- Lower cost of living
- Real estate less expensive
- Lower taxes
- Cultural and recreational activities
- Quality of healthcare
- Telecommunications

South of the Border – Down Mexico Way

This song is being sung by U.S. seniors heading south to capture less expensive housing and for their increasing health-care requirements. Living in another country may be daunting for some, but the idea of a mountain lake region brimming over with 40,000 to 80,000 American and European expatriates, along with a mild climate, is appealing to many.

- Nursing care costs in Mexico are much more affordable than in the U.S. making this move very appealing to Baby Boomers
- There are only 288 nursing-care facilities in Mexico, compared to over 9,000 in the USA
- The average costs for a private room in a Mexican nursing facility runs $18 to $50 per day compared to the U.S price of $206 (based on a 2006 MetLife insurance figure)
- One can also live in a studio apartment for $550 month which provides three meals a day, laundry and cleaning services, and 24-hour nursing care
- Cost of living is extremely appealing and the Mexican Social Security Institute (IMSS) provides full medical coverage to Americans for clinic and hospital costs. Medical coverage costs about $140 per year

There are downsides to living in Mexico, however, with little or lax government regulations.

- Drug cartels have created an unsafe criminal environment in certain areas
- Some nursing facilities suddenly go bankrupt, forcing people to find another
- Not all of the nursing facilities are class A
- The Mexican government doesn't have strict codes so many of the facilities are not monitored and two out of eight do not have State Health Department Licenses
- Medicaid, Medicare, Department of Veteran Affairs and many U.S. insurance companies will not cover any medical costs if you live in Mexico; in order to receive benefits from these U.S. governmental organizations, you would have to return to the U.S. for your medical care

As more retirement and nursing communities crop up in places like Lake Chapala, Ensenada, Rosarita, Puerto Vallarta, Monterrey and San Miguel de Allende, other homes have been forced to close due to poor management or unsanitary conditions. There is a bright future for increased and improved home-care facilities in Mexico. At the University of Texas in Austin, a forum made up of hospital administrators, insurance developers and policymakers convened to discuss the future of health care facilities in Mexico. Tijuana's Economic Development Council is asking the Mexican government to provide more federal funding to build more retirement facilities in Mexico. So, if "south of the border," Mexican cuisine, low-cost healthcare and affordable living are calling you, check it out. You may just discover a new life.

Other Countries to Consider

- Panama
- Belize
- Costa Rica
- Ecuador
- Central America
- Argentina
- Thailand
- Greece
- Portugal

Important Considerations

- Cost of Living
- Health Care
- Country national healthcare system
- Hospital care
- Healthcare
- Safety and crime rates
- Taxes
- Paying U.S. taxes
- Paying foreign taxes

- Senior benefits
- Collecting your social security
- Banking
- Visas
- Immigration details
- Residency requirements
- Buying real estate

Nine out of ten retired people over age 60 wind up staying right where they are. This is according to a verified AARP study: *Aging, Migration and Local Communities: The Views of 60+ Residents and Local Community Leaders.* Those who do move usually seek a warmer climate or move to be closer to family. Then there are those who never move (19%) and those who simply like their home and want to stay (14%). Those who relocate seem more satisfied with change when they are seeking a more affordable cost of living, less pollution, and new friends.

No matter where retirees reside and how they choose to live, we find that many "elders" of our society contribute their years of wisdom in their communities in a myriad of worthwhile ways.

> *"We have every reason to look forward into the future with hope and excitement. Fear nothing and no one. Work honestly. Be good, be happy. And remember that each of you is unique, your soul your own, irreplaceable, and individual in the miracle of your mortal frame."*
>
> ~ PEARL BUCK

Take Care of Health Care

Is the USA Social Security Secure?

Many Baby Boomers in the U.S. are relying on the government to help provide some income through social security beginning in their 60s. After all, Americans have paid up to 15% of their income toward supporting the Social Security system during their working years. However, Social Security is currently able to pay out funds that will put the recipients at or below poverty level if the only source of income. According to Dr. Olivia Mitchell of the Wharton School of Finance, Social Security is $11 trillion under-funded through 2017. By 2042, based on current statistics, the Social Security system will not be funded at all—it will be broke.

There are currently more than 77 million Baby Boomers in America (born 1946-1964) looking at 20 to 30 years of retirement, and having a longer life expectancy. Many of them hope to retire at age 62, the earliest age at which U.S. citizens can begin to receive Social Security benefits; however the qualifying age is rising to 67. In 1935, the year Social Security was founded, life expectancy was 70 years. It was assumed that people would retire at age 65, thereby requiring only five years of support from the Social Security system. The system was never designed or originally funded to cover 28 years of retirement.

Boomers Healthcare Challenges

Boomers want to be fit and healthy, and they are increasingly taking small steps to improve their well-being, primarily by eating healthy. But they still remain the most overweight age group in our nation. The latest data reveal that they find it tough to cut down on the bad stuff (e.g., alcohol and tobacco) and they exercise less.

Based on these habits, it is likely Boomers will continue to be heavily dependent on health care, the escalating cost of which is their leading source of stress. But, in large part because of a likely sharp increase in health care costs, the growth in consumption of medical products and services may be about to slow. With health care accounting for only about 5% of Boomers' expenditures, many employers believe there is still plenty of room for households to pay more for medical coverage. The catalyst for employees paying more could well be the Medicare Prescription Drug, Improvement and Modernization Act of 2003, which went beyond assisting seniors with prescription drugs and contained many other provisions that have wide-ranging implications for the entire health industry. A key provision of the Act is the establishment of health savings accounts (HSAS) which will likely have profound implications for both employees and retirees. In effect, an HSA is to healthcare what a 401(k) is to retirement savings.

Medicare

Medicare and Medicaid are both government-sponsored health plans. Medicare is primarily for 46 million seniors and disabled people with an annual cost of $500 billion. If you or your spouse has worked at least 10 years and are receiving or eligible to receive Social Security benefits, you are eligible to receive Medicare at age 65. When you retire, your employer-sponsored medical coverage will cease. If you do not have the resources to continue private medical insurance coverage, the government has designed Medicare and Medicaid to fill the gap. Three months prior to your 65th birthday you will receive an enrollment package to be filled out and returned.

Medicare's obligation to future retirees is currently underfunded by a staggering $62 trillion. Americans are currently paying 2.9% of their incomes in taxes to support Medicare. 61% of Americans support raising Medicare taxes in order to cover their benefits. Without intervention, the system of funding could unravel long before (our) grandchildren are eligible for benefits. In two decades Medicare will be covering over 80 million of the last Baby Boomers reaching 65 years of age.

An Overview of USA Medicare/Medicaid Provisions

Medicare - Part A Covers

- Hospital insurance is automatically provided at age 65 at no additional cost

Part B is an Elective Option.

- You will pay a fee (currently $96.50 per month for those earning less than $85,000 per year), but subject to annual change
- Covers doctor's visits, outpatient hospital care, ambulance services, rehabilitation therapy, medical tests, and some medical equipment

Medicare Part C Provides

- Option of receiving benefits through private health-insurance plans

Part D is a Relatively New Program Initiated in 2006

• Provides prescription drug coverage offered through various private insurance companies

These programs need to be carefully reviewed, as they vary widely in cost and coverage and also vary according to the part of the country in which you reside. The cost of prescription drugs can overwhelm people's pocketbooks; this program was designed to help pay some of these costs.

Medicaid

This program is designed to assist Americans needing help with their medical bills, regardless of age. On average, a person cannot earn more than $525 per month and can have no more than $1,500 in assets to qualify for Medicaid. For couples, the numbers change to $904 and $2,250 respectively.

Hospice

Hospice is truly an incredibly caring organization. When they came into my brother's home during our sister's last days, they supported us each day with a gentle and compassionate approach. They were there for less than a week and having them there during the late night hours helped us to step away for a short time and renew ourselves. After Pat died, the staff said how our team effort was inspirational to them. They shared that so many families are discomfited and ill at ease at the experience of seeing a loved one preparing to die. They leave it up to the Hospice team to handle everything. Our mutual desire was to be totally present for our sister. We played music and talked to her, even though toward the end she wasn't able to communicate. She was adamant regarding staying with us rather than being admitted to a hospital. Our loving efforts, and those of the Hospice workers, hopefully made her last days easier.

One out of three Americans call upon Hospice when a member of their family may have six months or less to live. There are organizations around the world. Hospice provides comfort in a home setting for the terminally ill. A support team may include a physician, a nurse, a home health aide, a social worker, a chaplain and a volunteer. One can contact Hospice for an international directory of Hospice organizations.

Right to Die

I am grateful that none of my family members has suffered a coma or has been hooked up to life support systems for long periods of time. They had the finances to live in their homes, have live-in help, and pay doctor and hospital bills. I read once that dying in ones sleep used to be more the norm and the best and most natural way to die. My grandmother Jennie passed in her sleep. Morality, religion and laws support the stance that euthanasia should be treated as a crime. At this time there are only two U.S. states that permit a right to die provision: Washington and Oregon. The World Federation of Right to Die Societies supports a person deciding when he or she wishes to die. Belgium, Netherlands, Switzerland, Luxembourg all support a final exit network.

> *"Death is nothing at all. It does not count. I have only slipped away into the next room. Nothing has happened. Everything remains exactly as it was. I am I, and you are you, and the old life that we lived so fondly together is untouched, unchanged. Whatever we were to each other; that we are still. Call me by the old familiar name. Speak of me in the easy way, which you always used. Put no difference into your tone. Wear no forced air of solemnity or sorrow. Laugh as we always laughed at the little jokes that we enjoyed together. Play, smile, think of me, and pray for me. Let my name be ever the household word that it always was. Let it be spoken without an effort, without the ghost of a shadow upon it. Life means all that it ever meant. It is the same as it ever was. There is absolute and unbroken continuity. What is death but a negligible accident? Why should I be out of mind because I am out of sight? I am but waiting for you, for an interval, somewhere very near, just around the corner. All is well."*

> *- HENRY SCOTT HOLLAND*

Costly Health Insurance

The U.S. has the most expensive healthcare in the world. Many people over 50 pay thousands of dollars a year in health insurance premiums alone. There are currently over 50 million uninsured people in the U.S. When you reach age 65 and qualify for Medicare coverage, you will no doubt still have out-of-pocket medical expenses. According to Fidelity Investments, if you are 40 years of age, you should begin to save $200,000 for your health care needs age 40 on, and that number can rise to $425,000 by the time you retire at age 65.

The Broken American Health Care System

In the USA, those age 65 and beyond are increasing twice as fast as the remainder of the population (U.S. Census Bureau). This is putting a tremendous strain on government health spending which is currently over $1.5 trillion. Diabetes has increased 45% within the last 20 years while heart disease, cancer and strokes have declined. Currently President Obama's health cabinet has many challenges ahead in providing less expensive health care to the aging. Hopefully within his term of office (through 2012), progressive changes can be implemented to help the increasing number of Baby Boomers and older people receive healthcare that doesn't financially overwhelm them. No other healthcare system in the world has medical bankruptcy, but in this country, over 700,000 medical bankruptcies were reported in 2010 alone.

Americans who are underinsured or uninsured currently number over 50 million. In 2009 over 4.5 million Americans lost jobs during the recession, and many continue to lose employment to this day. Americans also lost their health insurance coverage within an 18-month coverage period. Because the full premium has to be paid by the employee once they are no longer employed, 90% have chosen not to continue their job-related insurance plans. Add to this the fact that insurance companies, for their own internal policy reasons, often offer bonuses to their employees who deny certain claims or rescind health contracts. Seeking an alternative plan can be tricky, however; especially if you have a pre-existing condition or have a common ailment which could even be defined as taking a medication such as Prozac to help through temporary trying emotional times in your life. High deductibles and having to pay up to 40% of the cost of hospitalization forces many to put off needed surgery. If you lived in another country, chances are you would have your operation.

Health insurance troubles also trickle down to the younger generation. Full-time students are usually covered through their parents' health insurance policy. However, it becomes a different story when they graduate and go out on their own. They have to seek their own health coverage or sign up for a plan through their employer, if offered

President Obama's 2009 Health Reform Bill is in danger of being changed dramatically with the 2011 Republican majority in Congress. His healthcare reform was intended to propel the U.S. health care system in a more positive direction. In March 2009, the President invited doctors and insurance companies to the White House to discuss reform. Insurance companies and doctors agreed to consider the proposed changes. Former President Clinton tried to amend the insurance industry in the early 1990's; however, not much changed. The new reform bill proposes that every American would be Insured and the lower income population would be subsidized. This reform is being hotly debated in Congress, and may ultimately be decided in the U.S. Supreme Court.

America's higher medical processing fees, if cut in half, would be comparable to the costs in Taiwan or Canada. With lower costs, more of the uninsured can be covered. If more people were insured, they might receive the care they needed and 20,000 lives could be saved each year. Fees include physicians, hospital charges and services. European countries study new medical technologies to determine which methods bring benefits or profits. The U.S. does not.

There are five states which mandate health insurance: Massachusetts, Vermont, New York, New Jersey and Maine. The premiums are costly, with Massachusetts having the highest medical insurance costs in the country. These costs could go down if the Reform Bill passes, however.

The government Medicare and Medicaid system and private insurance companies makes it more complicated, however. The U.S. has a $2.2 trillion health industry which is made up of medical people, lobbyists, hospitals and patient care—many who complain they are already underpaid or cannot operate on less. So it may come down to a change of mind that less is more in order for the new healthcare reform to happen. The time is ripe to have health care reform in the U.S. Along with health reform, preventive measures must also be taken. President Obama has stressed how important it is to take responsibility for our individual health in order to help prevent debilitating diseases. He has also included some policies for this. Alternative and preventative medicine is not covered by many insurance policies. Double blind clinical studies for integrative medicine are barely considered in allopathic medicine. And yet a massive amount of prescription drugs are written by physicians. There are no double blind studies for that.

So how does one know the effect of ingesting multiple medications? My grandparents' cabinet was overflowing with prescribed pharmaceutical drugs. My mother received gold and cortisone injections along with her prescribed medicine for years. Growing up in a home full of medicine I began to question the detrimental effects, not to mention the cost. I turned toward more wholistic approaches for myself and my family. I encourage you to further explore the health benefits of complementary medicine.

Tooth Care Truth in the USA

An estimated 108 million Americans do not carry dental insurance. Having regular checkups and maintaining healthy teeth and gums not only saves our teeth, but helps to ward off certain diseases of the body including heart disease.

There are insurance options for dental insurance although they don't cover all dental procedures.

- AARP offers dental insurance through Delta Dental which operates like an HMO. In other words, they provide a national list of dentists under their plan, and you must use one of these dentists to be covered

- Care Credit is a charge card to be used for dental procedures; one needs to use a dentist on their list and apply for a certain amount of credit; they provide an interest free period after which there is a high interest fee applied on the remaining balance

- In order to cut costs, some people go to a local dental college where supervised students do the work at considerably lower cost

- Some go to Mexico for treatment

If any of these ideas are not an option for you, it would be wise to research different policies, especially if you are self-employed or if your employer doesn't provide dental insurance.

Shopping for Pharmaceuticals

In recent years, Americans—many of them older—have spent between $500 million and $1 billion annually on prescription medicines coming from Canada, where brand-name drugs, including those made by U.S. companies, are often much cheaper than the same medication purchased in the U.S. Although cross-border shipments of medications have been illegal for some time, authorities did little to stop the practice until late in 2004. At that time, the Department of Homeland Security began a crackdown on drugs being shipped into this country from Canada. By November 2005, the Department of Homeland Security's Customs and Border protection had seized over 39,000 packages of Canadian drugs coming into the United States. Recently, due largely to the hue and cry from retirees and various congressmen and women, DHS has backed off this policy somewhat. However, before ordering prescription drugs from Canada or elsewhere, it would be wise to check the law and current enforcement policy. Refer to the resource section at the back of the book.

What America's Healthcare Could Learn From Five Other Countries

The United States has been rated 37th in the world for fairness and quality of healthcare by the World Health Organization (WHO). We are a nation regulated by the pharmaceutical and medical industries. Until we have a leader of this country who doesn't have deep involvement with the special interests groups that support those institutions, we as seniors will continue to be at the mercy of accelerated medical costs and limited healthcare options which I strongly believe should include preventative medicine like acupuncture, Chinese medicine, chiropractors and massage therapists. This also includes professionals who are interested in teaching people how to have healthier lifestyles through preventative measures and thus eliminating many diseases which older people are susceptible to.

Healthcare around our World

I watched a Public Broadcasting Program, *Sick Around the World* which discusses other countries' healthcare reforms. This program is educational and informative, although certainly not perfect. Perhaps the U.S. can learn lessons from other parts of the world and incorporate progressive changes in our especially flawed healthcare system.

United Kingdom

The British are high on complementary medicine and herbs. If it's good enough for the Queen and her family, it must be great for the common people too. The Brits pay for their healthcare coverage through taxes which still equates to one-half of what Americans pay.

- The government owns the hospitals
- Doctors are government employees
- No insurance or medical bills
- No medical bankruptcy
- The wait for emergency primary care heart and hip surgeries is less than six months
- Patients have a choice which hospital they can go to
- Patients receive incentives to stay healthy

Japan

They are the second richest country in the world with a population of 130 million people. All Japanese are covered under a one payment system. Insurance companies are not allowed to make a profit. The downside is that 50% of Japanese hospitals experience financial difficulties.

- Highest life expectancy in the world
- Lowest infant mortality
- Government pays for the poor
- 8% of hospitals and physicians are private
- People can see any specialist of their choice
- No appointments necessary and may go often
- Longer hospital stays
- Twice the amount of hospital scans performed per capita compared to the U.S. and Britain
- Medical prices for procedures and drugs re-negotiated every two years
- MRI cost is $98 compared to $1,200 in the U.S.

- Hospital stay costs $10 per day, $90 for a 'private' room. (In Japan, a private room can contain up to 4 people)
- Medical machines are inexpensive to manufacture and are exported worldwide
- Doctors cannot get rich
- If a Japanese citizen loses his job they do not lose their insurance
- Employees pay half of the $280 month family health premium

Germany

In 1880 Chancellor Otto van Bismarck established healthcare reform which was named the Bismarck Plan. Germany is now the 3rd richest country in the world. Germany has private doctors and hospitals. Medical school is free although physicians do not receive high salaries compared to doctors in the U.S. With over 240 private insurance providers available they can compete for business but are not allowed to make a profit. Hospitals are not allowed to raise their prices. The government renegotiates hospital charges every year.

- All German people are offered healthcare
- The wealthy can elect to opt out and pay privately
- 90% of Germans are insured
- Healthcare includes medical, dental, optical and counseling
- Homeopathy and spa treatments included
- Short wait for doctor appointments
- People pay health premiums based on their personal incomes
- Workers can split their premiums with their employers 50%
- If they lose their job they do not lose their insurance coverage
- Pregnant women receive free healthcare

Some New Healthcare Options

You may be able to cut medical costs by going to a local medical school or finding a nurse practitioner. You might also want to explore TeleDoc (800-835-2362), which offers consultations by telephone. The initial registration fees are small, and there is a small monthly fee for these services. There are over 200 TeleDoc physicians listed in this network. Also, some retail stores and pharmacies have opened in-house clinics with a reasonable ($25 to $60) fee for an appointment.

Switzerland

Switzerland reformed their healthcare program in 1994. In this country of over 8 million, there is no medical bankruptcy. (U.S. has as many as 700,000 per year).

- The country pays for the poor
- Everyone is offered health insurance coverage and no one is turned down
- Pharmaceutical companies rated in the top 10 in the world
- Administrative costs are 5.5% compared to the U.S which can range between 20 to 30%
- Monthly family premiums cost $750
- Uninsured are required to pay their own medical bills

Taiwan

This island contains 23 million people and is considered wealthy. A healthcare program was initiated in 1995 by comparing the best health programs selected from 10 to 15 developed countries and choosing the best from each to incorporate into the Taiwan health reform. There is no medical bankruptcy, although the system is under strain due to rising medical costs.

- Free choice of doctors and no wait time for appointments
- All medical expenses are covered including traditional Chinese medicine
- National insurance system with one government provider
- Administrative costs are less than 2% per year
- Smart card assigned to each person with their health history recorded into a national system

Mixing foreign travel for pleasure, while seeking lower-cost medical services, seems to be growing in popularity. Many foreign hospitals have U.S. trained physicians and their rates are easily half that of similar care in the U.S., especially for orthopedics, dentistry, and plastic surgery. Some of the most popular countries providing lower-cost medical services are India, Africa, Thailand and Costa Rica. If you choose to explore these options, please check credentials carefully and, if possible, speak to someone who has been through the procedure you are seeking.

Forget Your Age: Live Now!

The Best Way to Live Your Life

Some of us made our riches early in life and retired at a young age to less stressful living, where we have a multitude of life choices to pick from. Some of us are still working toward the day we can hang up our hat and hope to have a generous nest egg tucked away, a comfortable pension, and other investments to assist in living out the remainder of our years in relative comfort. Some of us take what we have and head to areas of the world where our money stretches farther, the cost of living is lower, and we can settle into a comfortable home surrounding ourselves with like-minded people. If we have time on our hands, we may even start an on-line business or take on other part-time endeavors.

Some of us, however, do not have the luxury to stop working. Our Social Security payments will not cover our monthly living expenses and we do not have enough savings to live off of for the remainder of our lives; or we have too much debt to manage without a steady income. We feel we have no option other than to "play the hand that's been dealt."

Whichever position you find yourself in during this time of your life, there are always options to choose from. I have been single for over 25 years and have been self-employed most of my adult life. Thus my social security benefits are slimmer, I am not entitled to a pension, and my savings is clearly not enough for me to stop working. As dismal as that may sound to some and familiar to others, I have many blessings in my life. I have my health, family, beautiful places where I have lived, great friends and an everlasting presence of spiritual comfort, love and inner peace to sustain me in the most challenging times. I still have an alert mind and healthy body to continue creating more abundance in my life.

Aging may bring about risks to the mind and body such as memory loss, Alzheimer's or dementia, but ongoing research has found good reason to feel better about growing older.

According to Elkhonon Goldberg, professor of Neurology at New York University School of Medicine, aging does not always lead to loss and deterioration; it can also bring about rebirth and renewal. Professor Goldberg is the author of *The Wisdom Paradox: How Your Mind Can Grow Stronger as Your Brain Grows Older*. It seems that neuroplasticity, the ability to develop new neurons, is stimulated in people who keep their minds continually active as they age.

Goldberg cites Albert Einstein as a prime example. "When he wasn't working, he played the violin to keep his mind sharp." Goldberg emphasizes the importance of continually challenging our brains by "stepping out of our comfort zone and our repetitive routines." I now have a greater understanding of and appreciation for the long-term benefits of the board games, bridge, and other card games I played as a child and throughout my life.

> *"My grandmother started walking 5 miles a day when she was 60. Now she's 97 years old and we don't know where the heck she is!"*
>
> ~ *Ellen DeGeneres*

Sexuality

The adage "Use it or lose it" could be appropriate to many of us as we age. We may need to put more emphasis on creating sexual excitement. Our hormone production may have decreased but surely our desires to be held and satisfied are still hovering around us. True, it may take longer for us to become aroused and we may need more time to reach orgasm, but it is worth it to include this special intimacy in our lives. Common knowledge is that, along with the normal changes of aging, sometimes health conditions and medications play a part for men in achieving an erection. Diabetes, depression, high blood pressure and prostate problems can all play a role in diminished performance. Pre and post-menopausal symptoms in women may decrease sexual desires. Addiction to liquor, cigarettes or drugs certainly doesn't help, either. However, there are many natural herbal treatments available to help men and women increase their sexual desire and performance. Ask your health practitioner what he/she may recommend that wouldn't interfere with any medications you may presently be taking.

Healthy sexual activity has many benefits. Sex is great aerobic exercise—equivalent to walking up two flights of stairs. It can slow aging and perhaps make those eye wrinkles go away. The more sexual contact you have, the more your body will naturally produce more sex hormones which bolster immune systems and strengthen muscles and bones. There is a humorous true story about sex coming from a large (12-story!) German brothel that offers a 50% discount for seniors. The Director, Armin Lobscheid, says "All clients need to do is show some proof of age. There's plenty of demand and people have certainly been taking advantage of the offer. Older folks are more active than you think." This certainly sounds like more fun than senior movie or restaurant discounts.

If you don't have that special person to snuggle up next to, there is always a place in our hearts to express love to those close to us.

> *"Sex is fifty percent of what you got and fifty percent of what others think you got."*
> - SOPHIA LOREN

Is Retirement for You?

Many considerations come into play when people are contemplating when to retire; how much they have accumulated to help fund their retirement; if they have health benefits once they retire; and whether or not they are really ready to stop working.

Based on figures from 1995 and 2005, in a spread of 10 years the number of older people staying in the work force has actually increased; 82% of men ages 50 to 59 are still in the work force—no change from 10 years ago; 58% of men ages 60 to 64 are in the work force—a 5% increase; 70.1% of women ages 50 to 59 are still working—an increase of 5%; and 45% of women age 60 to 64 are working, a 7% increase over 10 years ago. Even in men and women age 65 and older, the percentage still actively in the work force is 19.8% and 11.5% respectively, a 3% increase for both sexes compared to the 1995 statistics. With the current world economic woes, more people will be employed in the later years to help supplement their retirement funds. Over half of Canadian citizens between ages 55 to 64 will stay employed because much of the middle class has an average net worth of less than $120,000, not enough to support them for the next 20 to 30 years.

In the United Kingdom the Daily Mail newspaper has suggested that the "Over 50's are being forced back to work to meet rising bills." They go on to say that "Poor pensions, sick partners, elderly parents and grown-up children who need financial support are common causes for working, rather than retiring."

> *"Twenty years from now, you will be more disappointed by the things you did not do than the things you did do. So, throw off the bowlines. Sail away from the safe harbor. Catch the trade winds in your sails. Explore, dream, discover."*
>
> ~ Mark Twain

Keep Inspired

It seems highly appropriate to address not only the over-fifty crowd and the Baby Boomers in this book, but the older generation as well. Living in Hawaii, I have witnessed phenomenal strength, energy, endurance and discipline during the world-famous "Ironman Triathlon." I have seen people in their 70's and 80's complete this grueling test of courage; some even in wheelchairs. I have asked myself, "What drives them to do this?" Perhaps it gives them a purpose and keeps them in the "game" of life. We are not all athletes of that superior ability; however, we are athletes of a different sort. We thrive on challenge, we continue to learn, and most of all, we believe we can continue to create a full life into our sunset years.

My 84-year-old-maternal grandfather surrounded himself with young people. He read voraciously and spoke several languages. He owned several businesses and never officially retired. He believed by doing these things he was invigorated and stimulated by active dialogue and the exchange of ideas and ideals with others, younger and older alike.

I recently read an article about an athlete named Erwin Jaskulski who held world records in track in the 95 to 99 and 100+ age groups. He passed away in 2006 at the age of 103. Even at 101, he was studying his technique to see how he could improve. He became an inspiration to others through his example of commitment and discipline. Not only an athlete, he pursued interests in music, philosophy, and could hold a lively discussion on a variety of subjects. His main philosophy was "to be happy and joyful in life."

Gilad of the Hawaiian TV show, "Gilad's Bodies in Motion," once saw

Jaskulski on the beach doing some incredible feats of exercise, standing on his head, running, doing push-ups, and thought Jasulski was amazing for a man in his 60's—only to discover he was 82 at the time! He and Jaskulski developed a lasting friendship.

The Remarkable Story of Jack LaLanne

In January 2011, Jack LaLanne passed away from pneumonia at age 96.. Almost up to the end of his life, Jack continued to follow his passion for healthy living. Jack LaLanne's dad died at age 50, but obviously Jack didn't believe genetics controlled longevity. He truly believed man could live to 150.

For more than a half century, the name Jack LaLanne had been synonymous with fitness, proper diet, and good health. He was often referred to as the "Godfather of Fitness." In 1934, at the age of 21, he opened the first modern health spa in Oakland, California and continued on to introduce exercise to television in 1951 on the popular *Jack LaLanne Show.*

Jack LaLanne's life was transformed at age 15 when he attended a lecture given by the health pioneer, Paul Bragg. At the time, Jack was sickly, hooked on sugar, and had a "junk-food" diet. From that moment he was changed forever.

Into his nineties, Jack continued to monitor his diet, exercise and supplements. His website sold his books and supplements, and before his death, he could be seen on television demonstrating and selling his juicer with the same trademark enthusiasm.

Jack's philosophy regarding healthy longevity was comprised of the following:

* Exercise and good nutrition
* Have a plan
* Too many people spend time watching television and drinking
* Get your priorities straight

"You have to work at longevity," he noted in an exclusive interview with Life Extension®. He believed that a sound program of physical fitness could lead to a productive and healthy life in our golden years. He recommended staying away from animal fats and processed foods, and reading food labels: if you cannot understand the ingredients, don't buy it.

- He worked out from 5:00 a.m. to 7:00 p.m. each day
- His meals were at 11:00 a.m. and 7:00 p.m.
- His morning meal consisted of 4 to 8 egg whites and 5 pieces of fresh fruit, often prepared with his juicer
- He and his wife ate out at restaurants that would prepare meals he requested; not all of us have this luxury, however, and can duplicate much of this in our own kitchens
- He ate salads comprised of many vegetables, with fish and turkey for protein
- He ate whole grains
- He avoided red meat and dairy products
- His supplements consisted of everything from A to Z including fish oil, cod liver oil, all of the vitamins, minerals, and enzymes

In his early years, Jack had to fight conventional medical wisdom which held that weightlifting would make athletes muscle-bound and inflexible, turn women into men, and put the elderly in an early grave. He was hopeful for the future because medical professionals now recognize the importance of daily exercise as part of a prescription for good health.

"Medical schools are now putting more emphasis on the value of nutrition and exercise, so future doctors can help people live longer," he noted. "Young doctors are now prescribing these things and the older ones are slowly realizing their importance. People need to change their patterns if they are going to increase their longevity. Even people in their eighties and nineties can benefit from exercise." Despite the considerable progress made in the last 60 years, LaLanne recognized that there was always room for improvement. "Even with all the scientific knowledge we have on the benefits of exercise, there are more fat people than ever," he noted with regret. "What we need is consumer education. People in the health field need to bind together to overcome the brainwashing that results from hawking junk food on TV."

"We have to start with the educational system, to teach our youth the right way to lead their lives. Kids are creatures of habit, so you have to get them to do the right thing and forget all that negative advertising they see on television. Until that's done, we won't make real headway in our campaign."

Up until his death at age 96, Jack LaLanne remained the eternal optimist. He had seen so much improvement since he started his crusade that he remained idealistic about the eventual triumph of the fitness lifestyle over a sedentary existence with its television, video games, junk food, and early death. "Nutrition and exercise should be an important part of everyone's life," he said. "Life should be a happy adventure, and to be happy you need to be healthy. Just take things one step at a time, and remember that everything you do takes energy to achieve. You need to plant the seeds and cultivate them well. Then you will reap the bountiful harvest of health and longevity."

> *"He laid the groundwork for others to have exercise programs, and now it has bloomed from that black and white program into a colorful enterprise."*
>
> ~ FORMER GOVERNOR ARNOLD SCHWARZENEGGER

Longevity in Other Lands

The Okinawa Centenarian Study (OSG) is a 25-year study based on solid evidence:

- People of Okinawa have a lower mortality and chronic disease rate compared to U.S., which ranks 18th
- They are lean and fit, they are strong boned, with healthy hormone levels, and have low rates of dementia, cancer, and cardiovascular disease
- Families care about their elders; they are not forgotten and shoved away in nursing homes until they die
- Stress is virtually non-existent
- Their diet consists of fish, vegetables, plenty of fresh water, and green tea
- They practice tai chi, dance, walk and garden; all natural and pleasurable forms of exercise

Other areas where the people live longer, healthier lives are:

- Andora (France), Macau (near China), San Marion (Italy), Singapore, Hong Kong, Japan, Sweden, Switzerland, and Guernsey (near the

English Channel).

• India is known to have the lowest level of Alzheimer's worldwide; the correlation may be their diet, which includes spices like turmeric which aids in anti-inflammatory responses in the body.

France

We've already mentioned the Mediterranean diet and its health benefits regarding Alzheimer's. Now from France, land of wine, cheese and rich sauces, there is another revelation in health and longevity. While Japan has the longest life expectancy at an average of 85.6 years, France averages 84 years, and increases three months a year. So by the turn of this century, the average life span for French women will be 95 and men 91 years of age. Compare Americans' average life expectancy at 80.1 years.

In 2006, more than 16,000 French hit the centenarian mark; that number has doubled in the last 7 years. According to the National Institute for Statistics and Economic Studies, there will be more than 150,000 centenarians in France by 2050. Longer life expectancy is spreading throughout Europe. Health care has improved along with lowered risks of drinking, smoking and accidents. The people who live in the southwest region of the Pyrenees in France may indulge in their local wines and rich foie gras from duck and goose liver, yet live longer than their fellow citizens who reside in northern areas. French women live a more relaxed life, eat and drink in moderation, stay active, laugh a lot and have a good time—an excellent example for all of us.

A French woman, Jeanne Calment, died in 1997 at the age of 122. She had the longest confirmed life span in the world. Not only did she live alone, but she took up fencing at age 85, continued to ride her bike, and appeared in the movie, *Vincent and Me* at age 114, making her the oldest actress in history. Jeanne met Vincent Van Gogh when she was 14, and found him to be "dirty, badly dressed and disagreeable." She claimed that giving up smoking at the "youthful" age of 117 attributed to her longevity.

The One-Hundred Year Mark

Centenarians, those who have reached the age of 100, currently number

50,454 in the United States alone. People who live 110 years, super centenarians, are estimated to number 450 worldwide. One in 50 women will live to be 100; for men, it is one in 200. Genetics play a strong factor, but also how people take care of themselves. A survey of healthy centenarians reveals that they credit their long life to their faith, a healthy diet, not smoking and strong family bonds. To avoid crisis care, many place self-care and healthcare high in their priorities. Only 4% of this group fear death.

Eric Plasker, D.C., author of *The 100 Year Lifestyle*, says that "being passionate about your life is the key to mastering your life." Look at the famous centenarian George Burns—smoking cigars nearly every day of his long life. I believe he must have been passionate about life; he certainly seemed to enjoy it to its fullest. L. Stephen Coles, M.D., cofounder of the Gerontology Research Group, states that "super centenarians escape from heart disease, cancer and stroke." So if we have made it that far, we must be doing something right.

The Old Wisdom
by Jane Goodall

When the night wind makes the pine trees creak
and the pale clouds glide across the dark sky,
Go out my child, go out and seek
Your soul: The Eternal I

For all the grasses rustling at your feet
And every flaming star that glitters high
above you, close up and meet
in you: The Eternal I

Yes, my child, go out into the world; walk slow
And silent, comprehending all, and by and by
Your soul, the Universe, will know
Itself: the Eternal I.

Afterword

Afoot and light-hearted
I take to the open road
Healthy, free, the world before me
The long brown path
Leading wherever I choose.

~ WALT WHITMAN

The last four years since Hawaii has been a grand exploration that has required me to retrain my mind, release stress, worry less, and live in the present moment by "going with the flow." Along with spontaneous adventures, I have been forced to take a look at my accumulated life-long patterns of resistance, control and fretting over what tomorrow may bring. Fortunately, I have had some excellent tools to assist me through these uncertain times. At a garage sale I bought *The Laws of Spirit* by Dan Millman. The story is about a man who meets a sage while on his mountain walk. The woman teaches him about compassion, patience, balance, choices, faith, integrity, and surrender. Relevant for all of our lives, I believe. I also have been listening to the teachings of Abraham channeled through Esther Hicks. Abraham frequently uses the metaphor of paddling your boat downstream instead of bucking the current. Abraham also teaches that what we believe, we become; thus the law of attraction.

My final surgery removed all the hardware and scar tissue from my wrist and arm, and I am so grateful to be on the mend. Physical therapy and a positive nature have helped make these challenging times a faint memory. I have not only re-discovered the wonders of my life but have been able to give myself a re-birth of youthful spontaneity and exuberance. I am enjoying and openly accepting where I am at this present moment along my path.

This book has been a labor of love which I tucked away in my mind for a very long time. I wrote it to share my life's experiences in health and mindfulness as well as guideposts for everyday living. The book shares many healthy ways to live through the foods we eat, our sense of purpose in life and how we can continually improve each day as we age. I hope that the information has been valuable in your path to wholeness through body, mind and spirit.

> *"There are two ways to live your life – one is as though nothing is a miracle, the other is as though everything is a miracle."*
>
> ~ ALBERT EINSTEIN

A healthy lifestyle can be quite simply described, and you've no doubt heard much of it before. It may not be so easy to do: Love yourself. Keep fit. Move and stretch regularly in a way that feels right for you. Eat the right foods in moderation. Love yourself. Avoid that which is possibly harmful. Stay focused in the present and think positive, peaceful thoughts. Learn to acknowledge and express all your emotions and quickly release them. Love yourself. Laugh a lot. Cultivate and honor your intuition. Give yourself the gift of regular solitude, preferably in a natural environment. Be honest—especially with yourself. Love yourself. Reduce stress through a practice of regular meditation, intentional loving, allowing, and detachment. Reconnect with your Creator, your higher self, by consciously cultivating faith, hope, trust, and surrender. Learn to live with reverence and gratitude. But most of all, love your self. Life always presents opportunities to reinvent ourselves. My grandchildren call me "Nonna"—Italian for grandmother. For now I have indeed become the Nonna who waits enthusiastically for the next voyage in my life. There are buckets of laughter with friends and family along with warm hugs from my many grandchildren.

> *"For a long time it seemed to me that life was about to begin. Real life. But there was always some obstacle in the way, something to be gotten through first, some unfinished business, time still to be served, a debt to be paid. At last it dawned on me that these obstacles were my life. This perspective has helped me to see there is no way to happiness. Happiness is the way. So treasure every moment you have and remember that time waits for no one. Happiness is a journey, not a destination."*
>
> ~ SOUZA

Recommended Resources

While the author has made every effort to provide accurate telephone numbers and Internet addresses at the time of publication, neither the publisher nor the author assume any responsibility for errors, or for changes that occur after publication. Further, neither the author nor publisher has any control over and does not assume any responsibility for third-party websites or their content.

Chapter 1

16 December 2006 issue of New Scientist BMJ, 2006; 333: 15–9

Science, 2001; 293: 1164–6

BBC Your Life in Their Hands series 1991

Acupuncture-Assisted Anesthesia: Narda G. Robinson, DO, DVM, MS 2007

Nutrition News 2003 VOL. XXV11, No I: The Mood Cure by Julia Ross MA

Archives of Neurology December 2005; Refer to the chapter on nutrition to find the chart

Medline Plus Exercise Your Brain and Body to Improve Memory. Reference: Johns Hopkins University Bloomberg School of Public Health

Massachusetts General Hospital

The Memory Prescription by Dr. Gary Small

The Aging Brain by Lawrence Whalley

AARP Bulletin online June 11, 2007

Frost & Sullivan's new report U.S. Alzheimer's Disease Medication Market

Alzheimer's Disease, Education and Referral Center at 1-800-438-4380. They can help you locate studies and answer your questions

Good Night: The Sleep Doctor's 4-Week Program to Better Sleep and Better Health by Dr. Michael Breus

Train Your Mind, Change Your Brain: How a New Science Reveals Our Extraordinary Potential to Transform Ourselves by Sharon Begley

Blink by Malcolm Gladwell

The Tipping Point by Malcolm Gladwell

The Biology Of Belief: Unleashing The Power Of Consciousness, Matter And Miracles by Bruce H. Lipton

Medicine, Mind, and Meaning: A psychiatrist's guide to treating the body, mind, and spirit by Eve A. Wood, M.D.

How We Choose To Be Happy by Rick Foster; ISBN: 039952990x

Big New Free Happy Unusual Life: Self Expression and Spiritual Practice for Those Who Have Time for Neither (02 Edition) by Nina Wise; ISBN: 0767910079

Authentic Happiness: Using the New Positive Psychology to Realize Your Potential for Lasting Fulfillment (Paperback) by Martin Seligman

The Living Matrix: The New Science of Healing DVD demonstrates how energy is as vital as our understanding of genetics in healing

Websites

www.sedona.com

www.jeanhouston.org/foundation

www.centerpoint.com

www.drwaynedyer.com

www.wakeuplaughing.com/ Swami Beyondananda

www.upliftprogram.com/depressionstats.html#statistics

www.umm.edu/altmed/ConsSupplements/Tyrosinecs.html

www.psychosomaticmedicine.org

www.alzfdn.org

www.nia.nih.gov/Alzheimer's/ResearchInformation/ClinicalTrials

www.researchandmarkets.com/research/02653b/u_s_alzheimers_d

www.drjilltaylor.com

Chapter 2

The Blue Zones: Lessons for Living Longer from the People Who've Lived the Longest by Dan Buettner

Thrive: Finding Happiness the Blue Zone Way by Dan Buettner

USA Today: Fit Smart by Jorge Cruise: Helpful Tips For Your Everyday Life

Walking: The Ultimate Exercise for Optimum Health (Audio CD) by Andrew Weil and Mark Fenton

Walk Away the Pounds: The Breakthrough 6-Week Program That Helps You Burn Fat, Tone Muscle, and Feel Great without Dieting by Leslie Sansone

Walking Magazine: The Complete Guide To Walking: for Health, Fitness, and Weight Loss

The New Yoga for Healthy Aging: Living Longer, Living Stronger and Loving Every Day by Suza Francina

Richard Hittleman's Yoga: 28 Day Exercise Plan by Richard Hittleman

Rodney Yee's *Yoga for Beginners* DVD by Rodney Yee

Kundalini Yoga with Gurmukh

Kundalini Yoga for Beginners and Beyond by Ravi Singh & Ana Brett

Kundalini Yoga to Detox & Distress by Maya Fiennes

The Everything Pilates Book by Amy Taylor Alpers and Rachel Taylor Segel

The Pilates Body by Brooke Siler

Kathy Smith's Pilates tapes provide really good instruction on the basics: Method-Precision Toning for the more advanced body

The Ph Miracle for Weight Loss By Dr. Robert Young

Jumping for Health by Dr. Morton Walker

Websites

www.walking.about.com

www.niadance.com

www.nqa.org

www.backrevolution.com

www.energycenter.com

www.amazon.com

www.patienteducation.stanford.edu/internet/healthyliving.html

www.alz.org

Bob Greene's books: www.onlinediets.biz/oprah/bobgreenebooks.htm

Suggested resource for fitness plans, health clubs, and senior activities: www.silversneakers.com/

For information on the Web about Pilates and how to find a certified instructor: www.thepilatescenter.com *or* www.thepilatesmethodalliance.com

Chapter 3

Food Rules by Michael Pollan

Don't Drink the Water by Lono A'o

Drinking Water Book by Colin Ingram

The Blue Death: Disease: Disaster and the Water We Drink. By Robert D Morris

The End of Overeating by David A Kessler, M.D.

Women, Food and God by Geneen Roth

Natures Field Insights on Inflammation by Steven H. Horne, RH Volume 22 No 33

Anti Inflammation Zone by Dr. Barry Sears

Eating for Beauty by David Wolfe

Eating for Beauty documentary: Woody Harrelson, Anthony Robbins and Aaron

Butler

Simply Raw: Reversing Diabetes in 30 Days

The Sunfood Diet Success System and Naked Chocolate by David Wolfe

Fats That Heal, Fats That Kill by Udo Erasmus, PhD

The PH Miracle for Diabetes: The Revolutionary Diet Plan for Type 1 and Type 2 Diabetics by Dr Robert O. Young

The Acid-Alkaline Food Guide: A Quick Reference to Foods & Their Effect on PH Levels by Susan E. Brown

Sugar Blues by William Dufty

There Is a Cure for Diabetes: The Tree of Life 21-Day+ Program by Gabriel Cousens

Rainbow Green Live Food Cuisine by Gabriel Cousens, M.D.

Delicious Living April 06 Jodi Helmer

Tjäderhane, L. and Larmas, M. A High Sucrose Diet Decreases the Mechanical Strength of Bones in Growing Rats. Journal of Nutrition. 1998:128:1807_1810.

The use of sorbitol- and xylitol-sweetened chewing gum in caries control – JAM Dental Assoc, Vol 137, No 2,90-196, Oral Care Report Vol. 13 No. 2, 2003

Vitamin Retailer: April 2006

The Miracle of Stevia by James May

Websites

www.mulitpureco.com – water filtration systems

www.bestfilters.com

www.phmiracleliving.com

www.drweil.com

www.flouridealert.com

www.grahamkerr.com

www.rawveganbooks.com

If you have concerns regarding the affects of fluoride, this is an excellent site which goes into greater depth regarding the pros and cons: www.flouridedebate.com

www.TheGreenGuide.com for updates on POPs in other farmed fish

www.mythbusters.com – regarding dioxins and microwave cooking

A wallet-size guide of the dirty dozen food list can be obtained from www.foodnews. org/reportcard.php

For more information on the Dirty Dozen, government regulatory issues and pesticide levels, go to www.foodnews.org or www.foodnews.org/pdf/EWG_pesticide.pdf

www.phmiracleliving.com/books.htm

To research which cooking pots and utensils are safer to use, go to http://environment.about.com/od/healthenvironment/a/safecookware.htm

www.organicconsumers.org/Toxic/safe-fish.cfm

www.mbayaq.org – click on Seafood Watch

kleankanteen.com sells one hundred percent recycled food grade stainless drinking containers for adults and children

Chapter 4

Comparative Guide to Nutritional Supplements by Lyle MacWilliam

Healthy Diet, Disease Prevention, and Longevity by Drs. Eberhard and Phyllis Kronhausen

How to Live Longer and Feel Better by Linus Pauling

The Vitamin D Solution by Michael F. Holick, PhD, M.D.

Life Extension Magazine September 2010: The Pioneer of Vitamin D Research

Lockwood, K., Moesgaard, S., Flokers, K., Partial and Complete Regression of Breast Cancer in Patients in Relation to Dosage of Coenzyme Q10: Biochemical and Biophysical Research Communications, Vol. 199, No. 3:1504-1508, 1994.

Peet M. Murphy Shaw j. Horrobin D.: Depletion of omega-3 fatty acids in red blood cell membranes of depressive patients. Biol Psychiatry. 1998 Mar; 1:43 (5):315-9

Maes M. Christophe A, Delanghe J Altamura C. Neels H. Meltzer HY: Lowered omega 3 polyunsaturated fatty acids in serum phospholipids and cholesteryl esters of depressed patients. Psychiatry Res. 1999 Mar 22:85(3):275-91

Dr. Susan Love's Menopause and Hormone Book by Susan Love, M.D.

AMA Journal; August 16, 2000

Herbal Healing Secrets for Women by Laurel Vukovic

LE Magazine: Rhoden, E.I. et al 2004; Schaeffer, E.M. et al 2004; Ebert T. et al 2005

Life Extension National Diagnostics, Inc. 1-800-208-3444

Life Extension Health Concerns (Online Magazine): "Male Hormone Restoration - Testosterone, Testosterone Levels, Testosterone Therapy"

Life Extension Health Concerns (Online Magazine) 2001: "Getting the Most from Exercise"

American Journal of Clinical Nutrition, January 2006

Eat, Drink and Be Healthy by Walter C. Willett, M.D.

The Dana-Farber Cancer Care Institute in Boston, MA

Memorial Sloan-Kettering Cancer Center, New York, NY

The Sidney Kimmel Comprehensive Cancer Center at John Hopkins in Baltimore, MD

The University of Texas M. D. Anderson Cancer Center in Houston, TX

American Society of Plastic Surgeons

The National Cancer Institute's page on clinical trials

Websites

www.newchapter.info – look under Herbal Therapeutics

www.cumc.columbia.edu/news/press_releases/zyflamend.html

www.prostate90.com

www.ajcn.org/cgi/content/abstract/84/2/419 - Published in the August, 2006 issue of the American Journal of Clinical Nutrition

www.newstarget.com/dairy_products.html

www.wildernessfamilynaturals.com

www.mcg.edu – The Clinical Microbiology Review October 2003

www.naturessunshine.com

www.acu-cell.com

www.lef.org Life Extension Foundation: excellent resource for clinical studies as well as supplements.

naturopathic.org or saliva.com

www.ClinicalTrials.gov – the US National Institute of Health's clinical trial website

www.eCancerTrials.com allows you to search for clinical trials by cancer type and cancer stage

Chapter 5

Healing Power of Sunlight and Vitamin D by Dr. Michael Holick

Life Extension Magazine August 2003: Fighting Back Against Skin Aging

Chinese Medicine for Beginners by Achim Eckert

You Don't Need Botox by Martha Lucas, PhD., and Denise Ellinger, L.Ac

6 Weeks to Sensational Skin by Dr. Loretta Ciraldo

The Healing Sun: Sunlight and Health in the 21st Century (Paperback) by Richard Hobday

Spa Directory by Susan Duckett (available on amazon.com)

American Society of Plastic Surgeons

BBC 4, October 2000

Institute of Pharmacology and Toxicology – University of Zurich, Switzerland Environmental Heath111 Perspectives 28 February 2001

Life Extension Magazine August 2003: Fighting Back Against Skin Aging

Websites

www.ewg.org/skindeep

www.MyChelleUSA.com

www.juicebeauty.com

www.emerita.com

www.jurlique.com

www.nvperriconemd.com

www.clarisonic.com

www.safecosmetics.org

www.gayot.com/lifestyle/spa/top10destinationspas.html
www.visiteuropeanspas.com/european-spas-association

Chapter 6

Inheritance Statistics: Federal Reserve Bank of Cleveland

The Coming Crunch: As U.S. Population Continues To Swell, Researchers Foresee Megacities, Crowded Coasts by June Kronholz; Wall Street Journal, October 13, 2006

Global Shift: How a World View is Transforming Humanity by Edmund J Bourne

Secrets of Simplicity by Mary Carlomag

EONS – a 50 plus media organization founded by Jeff Taylor of MONSTER.com

AARP Bulletin September 2006

The New Health Insurance Solution: How to Get Cheaper, Better Coverage without a Traditional Plan by Paul Zane Pilzer

Public Broadcasting Service (PBS) 'Frontline' by T.R. Reid: *Sick around the World*

Sicko (1907) Michael Moore's Movie Exposé on U.S Health Insurance. The documentary targets the major flaws in the American healthcare system.

Websites

www.turbosonicusa.com

www.michaelmoore.com

www.nccam.nih.gov National Institute of Health's National Center for Complementary and Alternative medicine

www.myss.com

www.elderhostel.org

www.ncpa.org/prs/rel/2004

www.aarp.org for more info go to Private Health Insurance Health Coverage Among Persons Age 50 Through 64

For additional information and guidance for the purchase of pharmaceuticals, check out these on-line resources:

www.pharmacychecker.com – For medications via mail order

www.medicarerights.org – discount drug cards and pharmacies, prescription assistance programs

www.crbestbuydrugs.org – A Consumer Report site to help compare drug options

www.aarp.org/comparedrugs – for cheapest and most reliable drugs

www.hospicenet.org

Chapter 7

The Joy of Sex and How to Be a Better Lover by William Campbell Douglass M.D.

The Wisdom Paradox: How Your Mind Can Grow Stronger as Your Brain Grows Older by Elkhonon Goldberg

Healthy at 100: the Scientifically Proven Secrets of the World's Healthiest and Longest Lived Peoples by John Robbins

Gazette Montreal Canada, Sept 2008

AARP Magazine November/December 2006

AARP Bulletin December 21, 2010

The 100 Year Lifestyle by Eric Plasker, D.C.

Websites

www.med.nyu.edu

http://psyphz.psych.wisc.edu

www.jacklalanne.com

www.okinawaprogram.com – National Geographic article on aging published in May 2005.

www.agewave.com

www.nationalgeographic.com/ngm/0511/feature1/index.html

www.Abraham-hicks.org

Miscellaneous Recommended Resources

Train Your Mind, Change Your Brain: How a New Science Reveals Our Extraordinary Potential to Transform Ourselves (Hardcover) by Sharon Begley

Blink and The Tipping Point by Malcolm Gladwell

The Biology Of Belief: Unleashing The Power Of Consciousness, Matter And Miracles (Hardcover) by Bruce H. Lipton

Medicine, Mind, and Meaning: A psychiatrist's guide to treating the body, mind, and spirit by Eve A. Wood, M.D.

How We Choose To Be Happy: by Rick Foster; ISBN: 039952990x

Big New Free Happy Unusual Life: Self Expression and Spiritual Practice for Those Who Have Time for Neither (02 Edition) by Nina Wise; ISBN: 0767910079

Authentic Happiness: Using the New Positive Psychology to Realize Your Potential for Lasting Fulfillment (Paperback): by Martin Seligman

www.wakeuplaughing.com/ Swami Beyondananda

The Living Matrix: The New Science of Healing: DVD. This film demonstrates how energy is as vital as our understanding of genetics in healing

www.sedona.com

www.jeanhouston.org/foundation

www.centerpoint.com

www.drwaynedyer.com

Acknowledgements

People have come into my life to help guide and support me. I call them "angels." I wish to express my heartfelt gratitude to those individuals who have contributed their talents to assist in this current book project.

Nigel Yorweith and Patricia Spadaro - your expertise in the publishing field helped to guide me through the initial stages of this book. Providing outlines, sources, and the right people made a tremendous difference for having this book come together in the right way.

Anne Barthel - Your editing style and outlines helped to clarify and smooth out the ragged edges of the written material. Your vision and development helped to create a more dynamic book.

Paul Bond - Through your artistic and creative talents, your exquisite layout and design work made this book come to life. It was a pleasure to collaborate with you once again.

Lynn Kelly - Many thanks for taking the manuscript into the pre final editorial corrections. You are a true master and yogi.

Susan Tinkle - We have collaborated for the last 15 years. Your edits are like your artwork, finely designed.

About the Author

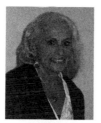 **Cynthia Olsen** {pen name} is the author of several books and a successful publisher. Ms Olsen began writing books on health in 1989. In 1990, her journey led her to create Kali Press, an enterprising publishing company committed to works addressing the full spectrum of life awareness with concentration on natural healing modalities. Over the next twelve years she delighted in the opportunity to assist other authors, research multiple books on complimentary health choices and to become a welcomed speaker regarding health and publishing.

In addition to her role as mother to her five children and her role as Nonna for her eight grandchildren, Cynthia is a lifelong supporter and exponent of holistic living. Cynthia's managerial experience allowed her to energetically advocate and support holistic living practices. Balancing all the demands she set in front of her, she also formed an import company in 1985, becoming a leader in introducing Australian Tea Tree Oil into the North American health scene. Her appetite for continued learning and healthy lifestyle choices has amassed a wealth of information, which she willingly shares through writing and speaking engagements.

Her book *Essiac: A Native Herbal Cancer Remedy* won the Small Press Book Award in 1997. As a result of her research into this remarkable herbal treatment, Ms. Olsen and Kali Press participated in a program to bring its benefits to the Second Mesa Pueblo of the Hopi Nation.

She has appeared on television, radio, and has addressed various conventions and meetings on health and natural living.

From her home in Colorado as well as her travel venues, she continues to actively pursue her varied interests in health, spirituality and joyful living. Ms. Olsen's new book *Looking Up: Seven Steps for a Healthy & Youthful Midlife and Beyond* has been a labor of love because of her passion for healthy aging beyond fifty. Ms Olsen's previous books have been translated into Spanish and German.

Ms Olsen has been a member of NNFA (Natural Nutritional Food Association), SOHO (Southern Health Organization), PMA (Publishers Marketing Association) and NFA (Natural Food Association).

Information and Order Page

(Ordering details on last page)

Essiac: A Native Herbal Cancer Remedy
Cynthia Olsen

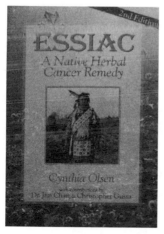

Winner of the Small Press Book Award in Medicine
The 2nd edition has been expanded to include case studies from Christopher Gussa, a clinical herbalist; plus an updated resource directory. This book gives a complete account of the recipe, the doses, and Essiac's uses. Also included are experiences of patients who have attained relief or regeneration from this remarkable herbal preparation.
144 pages, $12.50

"In November 1999, I was fighting prostate cancer and had a PSA (prostate specific antigen) reading of 17.9. I began to use the Essiac Herbals™ formula and in 4 months my PSA reading had dropped to .09. By December 2000 I was feeling great. The intense arthritis pain that I have endured has lessened, there is color in my skin, and my bowel movements are normal. I haven't felt this good in 25 years!"
~ D.W.

"This formula is a gift from the Ojibwa to all mankind, all races, anyone!"
~ OJIBWA MEDICINE MAN

Australian Tea Tree Oil First Aid Handbook: 101 plus Ways to Use Tea Tree Oil
Cynthia Olsen

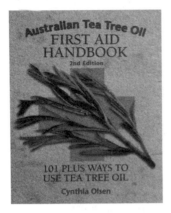

The second edition has been expanded to include more comprehensive skin uses for tea tree oil from head-to-toe. This convenient travel size book covers 101 plus ways to use tea tree oil. For nearly a century, Australian tea tree oil has been proven clinically effective for over 100 various skin conditions. Learn how to incorporate tea tree oil into your health and beauty care with this informative handbook.

96 pages, $6.95

"For topical infections, try tea tree oil, obtained from Melaleuca alternifolia. ..{It} is an excellent disinfectant, useful in first-aid kits for the home and when traveling."

-Andrew Weil, M.D.

Australian Tea Tree Oil Guide: First Aid Kit in a Bottle
Cynthia Olsen

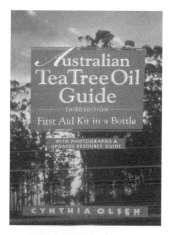

The 3rd Edition, Revised has been expanded to include photographs and an updated resource guide. Author/researcher Cynthia Olsen presents the most comprehensive book on Australian tea tree oil, known as the fantastic "first aid kit in a bottle." Follow the progress of this time-honored remedy from plantation to store shelf; includes chapters about tea tree oil for children, animals, testimonials, suggested uses, and clinical research.
144 pages, $9.95

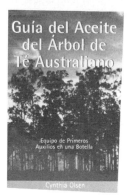

"This is an important book. It offers a concise and readable account of tea tree oil - one of nature's most versatile healing substances. This book is useful for consumers and the growing number of physicians and pharmacists becoming interested in natural medicine."

–MARK BLUMENTHAL, FOUNDER & DIRECTOR OF THE AMERICAN BOTANICAL COUNCIL

Don't Drink the Water (without reading this book)
Lono A'o

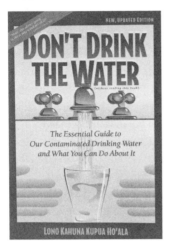

This is a complete resource guide to educate you on American public water systems, which are in crisis. Your tap water and your health are inseparable; high blood pressure, asthma, and ulcers can be relieved or prevented by drinking adequate amount of purified water.

Don't Drink the Water will help you decide which treatment system is best to have in your home. Find out why radon, fluoride and chlorine are detrimental for your health.

The author presents precise information you need to make intelligent decisions about the safety and treatment of your water. The vital information contained in Don't Drink the Water assists you in becoming active in one of the most important issues of our time. Learn what's really in your glass. **112 pages, $11.95**

"This is the most up-to-date and readable work I've seen on the subject... Study the advice on these pages and act on it!"

~ ANDREW WEIL, M.D.

Birth of the Blue: Australian Blue Cypress Oil

Cynthia Olsen

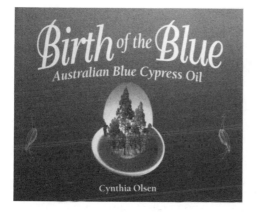

Birth of the Blue is the story of a recently discovered essential oil from Australia's Northern Cypress Pine – *Callitris intratropica*. This book contains a complete history of the discovery, research and development of Blue Cypress Oil including product development. This release contains illustrations, resources, maps, detailed testing and current standards. These books, along with products, were featured at the Sydney Summer Olympic Games in 2000.

88 pages, $7.95

"I have been using Australian Blue Cypress Oil in conjunction with my skin care services. Specifically, I have used the oil with micro dermabrasion treatments and acne extractions. I use a few drops of the pure oil in a soothing compress after these treatments and have found the inflammation and redness normally associated has been greatly reduced and in most cases eliminated. The smell is soothing and pleasing for both men and women. Most importantly, the results are consistent."

–Maryanne Garvin, Licensed Esthetician

Looking Up: Seven Steps for a Healthy & Youthful Midlife and Beyond

Cynthia Olsen

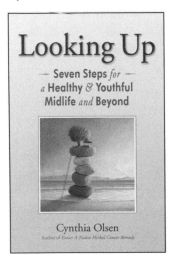

This ground-breaking book is for those seeking a healthier lifestyle, whether you are 40, 50, 60, or 100 years of age. The book shares guideposts for everyday living through the foods we eat, exercise, nutrition, living style, our sense of purpose, and how we can continually improve each day to bring more youthfulness and vitality into our lives. The seven keys presented by the author Cynthia Olsen communicate this vast knowledge to those seeking a more fulfilling physical, mental and spiritual way of life on one's path to well being.

Step One: How to cultivate a healthy mind and attitude

Step Two: How to improve your body through various exercises

Step Three: How to eat the right foods

Step Four: How to decide which supplements benefit your health

Step Five: How to keep your skin young and healthy

Step Six: How to take charge of your finances and understanding health care issues

Step Seven: How to discover the best ways to live your life

224 pages, $15.00

To order, please visit us at:

www.kalipress.com

Or contact us at:

Phone: 808-937-9793
Email: orders@kalipress.com

Kali Press
PO Box 5491
Eagle, CO 81631-5491